Eric Peters

The Pharmacogenetics of Antidepressant Response

Eric Peters

The Pharmacogenetics of Antidepressant Response

Moving towards Individualized Therapy - Improving Patient Outcomes through Optimization of Treatment Based on Genetic Makeup

VDM Verlag Dr. Müller

Imprint

Bibliographic information by the German National Library: The German National Library lists this publication at the German National Bibliography; detailed bibliographic information is available on the Internet at http://dnb.d-nb.de.
    Any brand names and product names mentioned in this book are subject to trademark, brand or patent protection and are trademarks or registered trademarks of their respective holders. The use of brand names, product names, common names, trade names, product descriptions etc. even without a particular marking in this works is in no way to be construed to mean that such names may be regarded as unrestricted in respect of trademark and brand protection legislation and could thus be used by anyone.

Cover image: www.purestockx.com ⸱

Publisher:
VDM Verlag Dr. Müller Aktiengesellschaft & Co. KG , Dudweiler Landstr. 125 a, 66123 Saarbrücken, Germany,
Phone +49 681 9100-698, Fax +49 681 9100-988,
Email: info@vdm-verlag.de

Zugl.: San Francisco, University of California at San Francisco, Diss., 2007

Produced in USA and UK by:
Lightning Source Inc., La Vergne, Tennessee, USA
Lightning Source UK Ltd., Milton Keynes, UK
BookSurge LLC, 5341 Dorchester Road, Suite 16, North Charleston, SC 29418, USA

ISBN: 978-3-8364-7055-1

ACKNOWLEDGEMENTS

Knowledge is priceless. Perhaps this is because the process of acquiring it is painfully slow - entire careers and countless hours of work have been performed in hopes of adding just small pieces to our fragmented understanding of the natural world. Frustrations and setbacks abound, as experiments fail and assays stop working when needed most. But the prospect of improving human health, advancing a field, or simply being the first to know something has a certain intrinsic appeal. What is clear is that knowledge cannot be pursued as a solo endeavor. I was fortunate to have the support of a tremendous group of colleagues, family and friends. Without them, I would have never made it through the process.

First and foremost, I would like to thank Steve Hamilton. His guidance is the reason my graduate school career had the bright spots that it did. He has taught me that science, at its very core, is not about a single experiment or laboratory technique. Instead, it is about the pursuit of knowledge, and to be a successful scientist one cannot succumb to tunnel vision. I've spent many engaging hours in his office discussing such varied topics as genetics, psychiatry, and religion, and he has always encouraged any curiosity or interest that I felt a need to discuss, no matter how irrelevant it was to my particular thesis project. He has also taught me the art of presenting science that is both exciting and accessible to the audience, which is an invaluable tool for any independent investigator. His commitment to science is an inspiration to me, as are his dedication to mentoring, patient care, and his family.

I would also like to thank Deanna Kroetz and Pui-Yan Kwok, my thesis committee, for their invaluable advice and insight. In addition to technical expertise, their guidance helped me focus my experiments on specific, attainable goals and

i

taught me the value of well thought out scientific inquiries. Also, Leslie Benet and David Glidden, who served on my qualification committee, taught me the importance of examining proposed research from several directions and disciplines.

I am lucky to be Steve's first graduate student, and as such I have witnessed several extraordinary people join his scientific team. Each has helped in some way on this project or making the lab a fun place to "work". In particular, Jeff Kraft, another graduate student in the lab, has been an important collaborator both in lab and out. Also, our basement neighbors the Genomics Core Facility, led by Elaine Carlson, have been incredible roommates and collaborators. Without their technical advice and skill, this project would have taken decades to complete.

The ups and downs of graduate school require people to lean on outside of the lab, and I have been fortunate to have many. Diversions are necessary to survive, and I've had the pleasure to have several partners in crime to pursue academic interests with: Ryan and Leslie Owen, Jeff (and Molly) Kraft, Kim Fife, Jason Gow, and Jim Shima. Most of all, I would like to thank Tom Urban, who I became friends with at our student orientation and have had entertaining times with ever since. I expect nothing less to occur in the future.

My greatest discovery in graduate school had nothing to do with science. I found my best friend, the person that would touch my very core. I met my wife, Leah, during my second year, and we have been inseparable since. Her sweet, kind spirit radiates from her everyday and I am blessed to be so close to it. She has had great patience with me, as afternoon forays into lab turned into midnight experiments, she was understanding and quite often by my side. She is my inspiration and motivation and her incredible strength of character is amazing to be near. The stories of our adventures and experiences together could fill several books, and these are what have shaped who I am today. She has taught me what is important in life; that we are guaranteed absolutely nothing but right now and so we had better make the most of it – thank you, Leah.

With Leah came the rest of her family whom accepted me from the beginning as one of their own. Her parents, Jimmy and Lodi Lagpacan, along with her sisters Leanna and Lara, brother-in-law Michael and niece Malia, have all shown us their support and thoughtfulness and trusted me with their beloved daughter, sister, and aunt. I'm also fortunate to have met Leah's extended family and shared great times with them.

My parents, Frederick and Sharon Peters, and my brother Jason and sister-in-law Kathy, have been a huge influence in my life. I'm confident that the reason I have a passion for science is because of my inquisitive and creative father, who would encourage any science fair project or question about our world. My mother encouraged me to read when I was young and would gladly take me to the library whenever I just had to have a new book on the animals of the African savanna or the ocean deep. I'm lucky to have been a graduate student and now to pursue new knowledge as a career. I would not have this chance without my parents, who always inspired and allowed me to further my education, even when it took me far from their home on the rolling plains of Northern Illinois. Even at a distance, it is a simple fact that, without their love and support, I would not have made it through graduate school and be where I am today. Thank you.

Eric James Peters

March, 2007

ABSTRACT

The Pharmacogenetics of Antidepressant Response

Eric J. Peters

Major depressive disorder is one of the most common and debilitating
psychiatric disorders. While psychopharmacological treatments exist, they are not
universally effective and can produce significant side effects in some patients. The
most common psychopharmacological agents used to treat major depression are the
selective serotonin reuptake inhibitors, or SSRIs. Often, these drugs take several
weeks to relieve depressive symptoms. If the initial therapy fails, other
antidepressants are often prescribed. This "trial and error" process creates a delay in
remission which can be frustrate the patient and lead to further decreased well-being.
Individualized therapy would have great clinical utility by identifying patients that are
likely to respond positively to SSRI therapy. The goal of the work described here is
to investigate the use of genetic markers for guiding treatment with SSRIs.

We utilized several complementary pharmacogenetic approaches and two
depressed populations treated with SSRIs. The first was a small (N=96) population
given fluoxetine, and the second was a large (N=1,953) population taking citalopram.
We used the fluoxetine population and a linkage disequilibrium mapping approach to
investigate variants in seven pharmacodynamic candidate genes for association to
response and specificity of response. Several variants in HTR2A and TPH1 were
associated with fluoxetine outcome. We then resequenced the coding region and 5'
conserved non-coding regions of these genes in the fluoxetine population in order to
uncover novel variation and additional tagging SNPs. These tagging SNPs were
genotyped in our citalopram population, and none of the SNPs were associated with

iv

clinical outcome. We then genotyped known, functional polymorphisms in relevant

pharmacokinetic genes for association to citalopram response and tolerance. Using a

two-stage study design, none of the variants were significantly associated with

outcome following citalopram treatment. We also utilized a whole genome

association study using over 590,000 SNPs from across the genome. Using a two-

stage study design, none of the most highly associated markers in the discovery

sample were also associated in the validation sample. Similar non-significant results

were obtained using multi-SNP decision trees. However, further genotyping is

necessary in the validation sample, as the most highly associated SNPs may not be the

most consistently associated.

TABLE OF CONTENTS

Chapter 2.

Linkage Disequilibrium Mapping of Variants in Pharmacodynamic Candidate

Genes for Association with Response to Fluoxetine

Chapter 3.

Sequencing of Pharmacodynamic Candidate Genes

Chapter 4.

Pharmacodynamic Candidate Gene Tagging SNP Selection and Association of

Tagging SNPs to Citalopram Response

Chapter 5.

Testing Functional Variation in Pharmacokinetic Genes for Association to

Citalopram Response and Tolerance

Chapter 6.

Whole Genome Association Study of Citalopram Remission and Tolerance

Chapter 7.

Summary and Future Directions

LIST OF TABLES

LIST OF FIGURES

Chapter 5.

Chapter 6.

CHAPTER 1

INTRODUCTION TO ANTIDEPRESSANT PHARMACOGENETICS

1.1 Major depressive disorder

1.1.1 Scope of disease. Major depression is one of the most common and disabling

psychiatric disorders (1). Depression is strongly associated with suicide, which is the

eleventh leading cause of death in the US overall, and the fourth leading cause of

death among 25-44 year olds (2;3). On average, treatment of depression costs

patients over $2000 per year and overall exacts an annual cost of more than $40

billion in the United States (4;5). Depression is a leading cause of disability

worldwide (2;6). The average age of onset for major depression is 25 years, and

depression is often chronic and characterized by recurrences throughout the lifespan,

with some estimates of recurrence as high as 85% (7). Major depressive disorder, as

defined in the DSM-IV, is characterized by at least two weeks of pervasively

depressed mood and/or diminished interest accompanied by vegetative and cognitive

symptoms, including sleep and appetite disturbances, psychomotor and energy

disturbances, cognitive changes and suicidal thoughts (8). Depression has high

comorbidity with other psychiatric disorders and substance abuse, and recent studies

suggest that depression may be an independent risk factor for some somatic disorders

such as heart disease and diabetes (9). Major depression affects 16% of the

population in the United States and the societal burden due to depression is

tremendous (1;10).

As with most psychiatric disorders, several different underlying etiologies are

likely to be responsible for the disease we label major depressive disorder.

Fortunately it appears that most patients with major depression respond to a variety of

1

treatments, including psychotherapies, psychotropic medications, and other somatic treatments such as electroconvulsive therapy (11). Psychopharmacological treatment is currently the most common and is expanding given the development of numerous classes of antidepressants over the past two decades (12). In particular, selective serotonin reuptake inhibitors (SSRIs) have become the most frequently prescribed antidepressant, due in part to their favorable safety profiles compared to older tricyclic antidepressants (13).

1.1.2 Response to antidepressants. While effective treatments for depression are available, it is clear that there is great clinical heterogeneity in response to antidepressants. The response rate to most antidepressants in clinical trials is on the order of 50-60%, with an even lower remission rate of 35-45% (14;15). Thus far, no clinical or demographic characteristic has been consistently associated with poor response to antidepressants (16). Nor have any reliable biological predictors been found to be associated with antidepressant response (17). Thus, patients who do not respond to first line antidepressant treatment often have to undergo additional trials with other antidepressants in order to achieve remission. This trial and error process is even more debilitating given the length of treatment required to gauge clinical effectiveness of antidepressants (typically 4 weeks or longer). Adverse effects of antidepressants also represent a substantial clinical problem, yet there is also currently no way to predict their occurrence. With the use of selective serotonin reuptake inhibitors (SSRIs) such as fluoxetine and citalopram, side effects such as nausea, sexual dysfunction, headache, sleep disturbance, tremor, and weight disturbances are commonly reported. One example of the magnitude of the problem is sexual side effects, which can occur in ~50% of those taking SSRIs. These adverse effects often result in non-compliance and discontinuation of treatment with no relief in depression

2

severity. A potentially devastating side effect involves increases in suicidal thinking among depressed patients, particularly adolescents, prescribed SSRIs (18). Other studies have shown no increased risk in self harm due to SSRI use and the controversial issue remains unresolved in the field (19).

1.2 Antidepressant pharmacogenetics

1.2.1 Pharmacogenetics overview. Pharmacogenetics, defined as the study of genetic variability between individuals in response to exogenous substances, as a field dates back to the late 1950s. The earliest modern pharmacogenetic discoveries of hereditary variation in drug response involved drugs such as succinylcholine, primaquine, and isoniazid. These classic studies set the stage for subsequent pharmacogenetic investigation, which currently focus on the genes that contribute to the pharmacokinetics (the actions of the body on drugs over a period of time) and pharmacodynamics (the biochemical and physiological effects of drugs and their mechanisms of action) of a particular drug (20). A great deal is known about the common inter-individual variation in Phase I (oxidation, reduction, or hydrolysis) and Phase II (conjugation) drug metabolizing enzymes, at both the enzymatic and DNA sequence levels (21). For example, an extensive catalog of functional variants and haplotype configurations in the genes encoding cytochrome P450 enzymes has been amassed (22). A major example of the success of pharmacogenetics involves the drug metabolizing enzyme, thiopurine methyltransferase (TPMT). Children who inherit two defective copies of this gene can experience fatal hematological side effects when administered 6-mercaptopurine, a chemotherapeutic agent used in pediatric leukemia, while patients with two normal copies of the gene for this enzyme require higher doses of the medication (23). Numerous examples exist for members of the

3

cytochrome P450 family of metabolic enzymes. Efforts at identifying genes involved in pharmacodynamics for particular medications have also been successful. Individual variations and haplotypes in the gene encoding for the type 2 β-adrenergic receptor have been found to correlate with response to β-agonists in the treatment of asthma (24). In addition, the dosing of warfarin, an anticoagulant with a narrow therapeutic index, was recently shown to be significantly influenced by the subject's genotype at a pharmacodynamic target of the drug (*VKORC1*) (25).

1.2.2 Pharmacogenetics of response to older antidepressants. Studies performed in the 1960s and 1970s revealed that upon repeated administration of one or another class of antidepressants, both response and non-response to antidepressant class were significantly concordant between family members (26;27). This finding has been replicated more recently in relatively small samples (28;29). The important role of cytochrome P450s in tricyclic antidepressant (TCA) metabolism is well-documented, and is reflected in the extensive work showing correlation between blood levels and response and toxicity, as well as the potential benefits of therapeutic drug monitoring for patient safety and reduced costs (30). Pharmacogenetic analysis guided by these observations revealed in one study that patients missing CYP2D6 could not be effectively treated with TCAs (31). In particular, persons experiencing adverse effects were more likely to be deficient for CYP2D6. This locus, which is highly polymorphic in the human population, has been suggested to account for 34% of the variation in plasma nortriptyline levels (32). Some authors recommend that pharmacogenetic considerations be taken into account with the use of TCAs, suggesting substantial dose reductions in persons with the "poor metabolizer" phenotype of CYP2D6 or CYP2C19 (33). Although commercial molecular diagnostics for CYP2D6 and CYP2C19 exist (e.g., AmpliChip CYP450 by Roche),

4

there is currently little evidence justifying their use in psychiatry. Some investigators have advocated the use of CYP genotyping for antidepressant therapy including SSRI treatment despite the lack of adequately powered studies showing benefits to clinical decision making (34;35).

1.2.3 Pharmacogenetics of SSRI response – pharmacodynamic genes. The current widespread use of SSRIs in depression along with recent advances in molecular genetics have resulted in a sizeable body of literature on SSRI pharmacogenetics (36). The majority of these studies focus on putative pharmacodynamic genes related to monoamine function, including the serotonin transporter (the molecular target for SSRIs), tryptophan hydroxylase 1, monoamine oxidase A, and the 1A and 2A serotonin receptors. These case-control studies as a whole examine a small number of polymorphic loci in these genes, and utilize fairly small sample sizes, ranging from 60-260 subjects.

In a sample of 222 Chinese patients with major depression, variants in the serotonin 1A receptor (*HTR1A*) were not associated with response to fluoxetine (37). Two SNP variants in the serotonin receptor 2A (*HTR2A*) gene (-1420A>G and 102T>C) were not associated with response to fluvoxamine or paroxetine in a sample of 443 patients (38). A variable number tandem repeat (VNTR) promoter polymorphism that influences the *in vitro* activity of the monoamine oxidase A (*MAOA*) gene also did not significantly influence SSRI response outcome in this study, or in a similar study conducted in Japan (38;39). There have been two studies investigating the role of an A218C polymorphism (rs1800532) in intron 7 of the tryptophan hydroxylase 1 gene (*TPH1*), both yielding significant associations to SSRI treatment response. In one study, the TPH*A/A genotype was associated with a slower response to fluvoxamine treatment only in patients not taking pindolol concomitantly (40). In another study by the same group, the TPH*A/A and TPH*A/C genotypes were associated with a poorer response to paroxetine treatment, with this association also not seen in the pindolol augmentation patients (41).

An Italian group has shown in a series of studies some evidence of an association between the long allele of a functional promoter polymorphism in the serotonin transporter and loosely defined depression, including cases of bipolar disorder in the depressed phase of the illness (40;42-44). Other groups have reported similar findings (45-47). These reports are of interest as this polymorphism is usually defined by the long and short alleles, with the long allele leading to increased in vitro transcription of the *SLC6A4* gene and serotonin uptake in cell lines (48). Additional notable findings in the pharmacogenetics of SSRI response have included associations to tryptophan hydroxylase (40), G protein β3 (49;50), angiotensin converting enzyme (51), and the glucocorticoid receptor FKBP5 (52). There has been little exploration of association between genetic variants in any of these genes and adverse events related to SSRI treatment. A small study showed that the short allele of the serotonin transporter promoter polymorphism was associated with the development of insomnia and agitation in a population of 36 outpatients (53). A study by Murphy *et al.* of 124 subjects with geriatric depression treated with the SSRI paroxetine showed that the genotype for a variant in the 2A serotonin receptor (*HTR2A*) predicted both greater rates of discontinuation and severity of adverse events (54).

1.2.4 Pharmacogenetics of SSRI response – pharmacokinetic genes. Previous studies investigating the relationship between SSRI medications and pharmacokinetic genes have been limited. The pharmacokinetics of many SSRIs, including citalopram, are affected by *CYP2D6* and *CYP2C19* genotype status, although there is no evidence regarding how plasma levels of citalopram influence clinical efficacy or tolerance

6

(55). In a study of 53 Chinese patients with major depression taking citalopram, *CYP2C19* genotype status was significantly associated with clearance of citalopram and the metabolic ratio of desmethylcitalopram to citalopram, but not associated with the primary clinical outcome of patient side effect burden (56). In the study by Murphy *et al.* cited above, they reported no significant influence of *CYP2D6* genotype status on paroxetine tolerance. Another study reported, in a sample of 100 depressed Japanese subjects, a gene by gene interaction between patient genotype at a variant in the *HTR2A* receptor and *CYP2D6* genotype status that significantly influenced risk of developing gastrointestinal side effects (57).

1.3 Genomics and association mapping

1.3.1 Overview. The effort to sequence the human genome has dramatically altered the potential impact of pharmacogenetics on human health. The vast majority of human genes have now been localized and annotated, although the biological function of many of these genes is unknown (58;59). One offshoot of this endeavor has been the discovery of the incredible level of sequence diversity between humans, largely in the form of single nucleotide polymorphisms (SNPs). SNPs are the most abundant type of DNA variation with over 12 million individual variants having already been identified and referenced at dbSNP, the SNP database hosted by the National Center for Biotechnology Information in collaboration with the NHGRI (http://www.ncbi.nlm.nih.gov). Single nucleotide polymorphisms have come under intense scrutiny as effective markers for genetic studies, partly out of their abundance, but also due to the development of efficient and inexpensive methodologies for assaying SNPs (60). Pharmacogenetics can now be broadened to "pharmacogenomics" in the context of the Human Genome Project, with our new annotated knowledge of genes, proteins, and SNPs allowing a more general analysis of the many different genes that determine drug behavior or even of the majority of the genes in the genome. The availability of other vertebrate genomes will aid in the identification of conserved non-coding elements that could have important developmental and regulatory consequences if they contain variation (61). Along similar lines, additional primate genomes (e.g., chimpanzee, gorilla, rhesus) will allow the identification of more subtle primate lineage-specific genetic elements that may be missed with more distant evolutionary comparisons (62).

1.3.2 Genetic association studies. Pharmacogenetic phenotypes are complex traits with contributions from pharmacodynamic genetic variants (transporters, receptors), pharmacokinetic genetic variants (absorption, metabolism, elimination), and environmental exposures. Given the genetic complexity of antidepressant response, the most powerful strategy for determining these genetic factors would be through use of an association study, also termed linkage disequilibrium (LD) mapping (63). In LD mapping, unobserved historical recombinations in an outbred population are used to identify disease genes by exploiting the physical proximity between a susceptibility gene and a marker locus (64). LD mapping thus assumes that some proportion of the cases have a common ancestor who had the disease-associated variation. The individuals who share this variation are also likely to share alleles at sites neighboring the actual disease locus due to linkage disequilibrium (65). The main advantage of this approach rests on the statistical power derived from the ability to collect substantial numbers of unrelated cases and controls (66). A number of interacting factors influence the likelihood of success in LD mapping designs, including the effect size of the trait variant, frequencies of marker and trait alleles, as well as LD relationships (67). Family based studies, while an attractive approach in disease mapping studies, are difficult to efficiently design and conduct in pharmacogenetic studies, given the low likelihood that an extended pedigree would have sufficient numbers of members treated with the same medication.

A disadvantage of LD mapping is the reliance on the assumption that common disorders are caused by high population frequency variants, which is known as the common disease-common variant hypothesis (CDCV) (68;69). This assumption is useful for LD mapping, since rare alleles (which are "newer") generally do not have significant LD (based on the r^2 measure) with neighboring alleles. Unless the actual causative rare allele is genotyped, it will generally not be captured by LD mapping. One potential way to circumvent this limitation of LD mapping is to use haplotypic (chromosomal configuration of several closely linked alleles) testing in order to "tag" rare alleles that were not genotyped. While haplotype testing can help capture rare SNPs and has other potential advantages, the utility and interpretation of haplotypic mapping remains controversial (70). The CDCV hypothesis states that common alleles, each contribute by themselves very small increases in risk (i.e., odds ratios from 1.5 - 2.5 for single alleles), but when combined and interacting with each other can determine the overall genetic risk for an individual (71). This underpinning for complex genetic phenotypes is not universally accepted, and an alternative framework known as the common disease rare variant (CDRV) hypothesis has been proposed. This hypothesis states that for any given complex phenotype several (on the order of 100s – 1,000s) of rare variants exist in different genes and pathways that each are individually sufficient to cause the trait (72;73). This model is similar to the molecular basis of most known Mendelian disorders, modified for more common, complex phenotypes. Unfortunately, using outbred populations it is difficult to collect enough samples to have adequate power to detect extremely rare variants

(<0.01 minor allele frequency) and family based studies are often not practical in pharmacogenetics. Furthermore, since the population attributable risk of rare variants will be low, they may have limited utility as diagnostic tests. In any case, a complicated matrix of rare and common variants are likely to play roles in pharmacogenetic phenotypes, even within the same gene (74).

1.3.3 Whole genome association studies. The vast majority of genetic association studies thus far have been candidate gene studies. Typically, candidate genes are chosen based on a biological hypothesis that connects the pathogenesis of the disease being studied with the function of the candidate gene. Often, theses studies are performed as "direct" association studies, meaning that a single DNA variant that is known to change the function of a gene product is genotyped in cases and controls. The major limitation of this direct approach is the necessity for some level of understanding of the biology of the gene and disease being studied. Often, for complex genetic disorders, we do not know *a priori* what genes will be involved. Candidate gene studies can also be performed as "indirect" association studies (LD mapping) by genotyping several markers within a gene and testing for association, relying on LD between the markers genotyped and the actual, unknown causal allele in order to uncover an association. An extension of LD mapping involves interrogating several thousands of markers across the entire genome and has been termed "whole genome association" (68). A major advantage of whole genome studies is that no understanding of the biological mechanism of the phenotype is required *a priori*, allowing susceptibility genes to be identified that were not considered candidate genes for the phenotype. To date only a few whole genome association studies have been published, and while there have been a few exceptional findings, results have been mixed and debate remains regarding the utility of these endeavors (75-78).

1.4 Challenges to association mapping

1.4.1 Phenotypic heterogeneity. There are several challenges to genetic association studies in either a candidate gene or whole genome context. As with all genetic studies, phenotypic heterogeneity is a concern. We can safely assume that the majority of clinical diagnoses, as has been shown with several types of cancer, are composed of different subtypes with distinct molecular mechanisms. Diagnostic techniques are limited in all fields of medicine and rarely identify the molecular causes underlying a disease or phenotype. This concern is even greater for psychiatric phenotypes, since these usually require the use of structured interviews or questionnaires for diagnosis. In our study, we attempted to limit phenotypic heterogeneity though the use of response pattern analysis (79;80). SSRI and other antidepressant medications have high placebo response rates, reaching 50% in some clinical trials. It has been shown that patients who have a delayed response (>2 week) to active medication and continue to maintain their response every week until week 12 ("specific responders") are more likely to relapse if blindly switched to placebo than patients displaying an early and inconsistent response ("non-specific responders") (80). Although the delayed response may not be a critical factor in determining true drug response, a sustained response seems to strongly predict specific response status (81). Thus, a subset of patients that appear to be responding to the medication are in fact having a placebo, or non-specific response. We performed association tests with these phenotypic subtypes in order to limit heterogeneity by accounting for non-specific response to SSRI medication.

11

1.4.2 Marker selection. Another obvious issue is which SNPs to genotype: with over 12 million known SNPs in the human genome and candidate genes often extending beyond 100 kb, current genotyping technologies prohibit complete ascertainment of all the SNPs within most candidate genes or all the SNPs in the human genome in reasonably sized clinical samples. Therefore, several groups have developed methods that exploit the LD between markers in order to reduce genotyping redundancy while maintaining the genetic diversity within a region. One of the computationally simplest methods attempts to select proxies, or "tagSNPs", in order to capture allelic information at other loci based solely on the pairwise r^2 measure of LD (82). Other methods select SNPs (haplotype tagging, or htSNPs) that capture the underlying haplotype structure (83;84). Still other methods select SNPs that, in combination, capture alleles at other, un-genotyped loci (85). There is no consensus in the field on which method has the most efficiency or power in association studies. For the candidate gene investigations performed in this study, we compared the efficiency and accuracy of several methods for selecting tagSNPs. For whole genome association studies the SNP marker panels are on fixed arrays in order to reduce production costs, therefore the investigator cannot change the SNPs to be genotyped. Current marker panels for whole genome studies have focused on gene-centric SNPs (ParAllele Biosciences), evenly spaced SNPs (Affymetrix), or used public resources like HapMap to select SNPs based on patterns of LD (Illumina). In our whole genome association study, we used a combination of approximately 40,000 gene-centric markers, 500,000 evenly spaced SNPs, and 50,000 SNPs chosen based on patterns of LD.

1.4.3 Multiple testing burden. Another challenge to association studies is the issue of multiple comparisons. Put another way, the likelihood of type I statistical error increases when one subjects a number of independent observations to the same significance criterion that would be used when considering a single event. In LD mapping, often several SNPs per gene are genotyped (or several thousand in whole genome studies), and some markers will reach statistical significance due to chance alone. One way to account for these multiple comparisons is to use a Bonferroni correction. For instance, if we set a $p<0.05$ Type I (α) error rate as our study-wide criteria for significance and interrogate 500 markers, the Bonferroni corrected criteria for significance would be $p<0.0001$ (α/N) for each individual SNP comparison. Bonferroni correction assumes the individual tests are independent of each other and clearly this is not the case for closely linked SNPs due to linkage disequilibrium, therefore this correction is generally considered overly conservative by geneticists (86). Permutation based empirical significance testing can allow for more accurate assessment of association in the presence of linkage disequilibrium, however computational constraints limit the application of some of these methods (87). An alternative method for controlling false positive rates is through use of a false discovery rate (FDR), or q-value (88). Instead of a simple p-value which can be interpreted as the probability that a test statistic as large or greater would occur by chance alone, a q-value is the proportion of tests above a threshold p-value that are likely false positives. A FDR threshold, which is not dependent on the actual number of tests performed, is determined from the observed p-value distribution and hence is adjustable to the amount of signal in the data and the number of false positives the investigator can tolerate in follow up studies. An additional method for controlling multiple comparisons is to use a split sample study design (89). With this method a study sample would be split into two roughly equal halves: a discovery set, in which all markers will be genotyped, and a replication set, in which only the markers that

13

reached the stated significance threshold in the discovery set are genotyped. Besides the cost-savings in terms of genotyping load this method also sidesteps some of the multiple testing issues since in the validation set only a subset of the total markers are tested, which requires less adjustment. However, by splitting the sample, we also greatly sacrifice power. We utilized a split sample design for our whole genome association study. There is still debate on which design is most powerful for whole genome association studies and it is likely that the underlying genetic mechanism, which is typically unknown, will determine the optimal study design (90).

1.4.4 Confounding due to population stratification. One of the main concerns for genetic association studies is population stratification. Indeed, fear of population stratification has caused family-based association tests to become quite popular in human genetics (91). Unfortunately, as stated above, pharmacogenetic studies generally cannot efficiently collect family based samples. Population stratification occurs when cases and controls have different allele frequencies attributable to diversity in background population that is unrelated to outcome status. In the work described in this thesis, the majority of markers investigated showed some level of differentiation in allele frequency based on self-reported race. For population stratification to have a detrimental effect on genetic association studies (i.e., to create confounding), there also must be a difference in baseline response (or disease) rates between the ancestry subgroups (92). In the STAR*D sample set, described in Chapters 4, 5, and 6, using self-reported race as a proxy for ancestry, several differences in response and tolerance existed across racial groups, indicating the need to adjust for population stratification in this sample. Uncorrected population stratification can cause false positive associations and can also mask true associations that occur within subpopulations (92). Several methods have been proposed to adjust and correct for population stratification. The simplest involves subdividing the clinical population based on self-reported race and testing for association within each substratum. It has been shown that self-reported race correlates well with genetic ancestry based on microsatellite and large-scale SNP genotyping (93;94). We used this method in our candidate gene studies in the STAR*D sample. Another method, known as genomic control (GC), uses unlinked markers across the genome to produce a scaling factor that is proportional to the degree of stratification (95). This scaling factor is then used to adjust the χ^2 value of individual SNP tests for differences in population background. The disadvantage of this method is that it applies the same scaling factor to all SNPs tested, when clearly some SNPs are more differentiated across populations than others. We used this GC procedure in our candidate gene studies in the fluoxetine sample, as described in Chapter 2. An alternative to the GC procedure is structured association, which also uses unlinked markers to detect stratification but attempts to define underlying subgroups within the stratified sample (96). After subpopulations are identified, association testing can then be performed within homogeneous subpopulations and additionally, a composite test statistic across all subpopulations can be calculated. A popular Markov chain Monte Carlo (MCMC) method for modeling population substructure is implemented in the program *structure*, which estimates the proportion of ancestry (Q) from "K" populations for each individual (97). Given that population subdivisions may be not occur as discrete clusters and the presumed levels of admixture in samples drawn from the United States, correctly choosing "K" is a difficult task. One way to select "K" is to run the model for several values of "K", and then use the estimates of the posterior probability of the model fit to select the most parsimonious value. In our whole genome association study described in Chapter 6, we used a structured association method to correct for population stratification within the STAR*D sample.

1.4.5 Detecting SNP interactions. Another major challenge in association studies of complex genetic diseases is the issue of interacting loci. An assumption of the CDCV hypothesis is that several loci, through interaction with each other and environmental factors, determine the individual's risk of response or adverse events from pharmacotherapy (98). A major limitation of detecting interaction loci is sample size. For average sized association studies (~100 cases and controls), even for two-way (SNP x SNP) interactions the cell sizes (number of individuals with a particular genotype combination) often are too small to have sufficient power to detect moderate effects. The problem of insufficient power becomes even greater when investigating uncommon SNPs or considering higher order (i.e., three-way) interactions. Furthermore, the number of statistical tests that result from interaction testing increases the need for large sample populations. For two-way (pairwise) testing, the number of pairwise tests (t) increases with the number of SNPs (n) in an exponential fashion ($t = 0.5n^2 - 0.5n$). In order to test all pairwise interactions in our whole genome study involving approximately 590,000 makers, we would have to perform 1.74×10^{11} statistical tests. Since most association studies to date have not been adequately powered to detect interactions, replicated interaction effects and validated methods for testing interactions are underdeveloped in the literature. One straightforward method for testing pairwise interaction is to use logistic regression modeling with an interaction term, and likelihood ratio testing to asses the significance of this model compared to the reduced model without the interaction term. We used logistic regression to test interactions in our candidate gene studies in the STAR*D sample. Inadequate power precluded testing for interactions in the

16

fluoxetine sample. While this method accommodates testing of small numbers of interactions, due to computational limitations, it is not applicable to whole genome data. For large scale datasets, tree-based methods such as recursive partitioning have been proposed (99). The main limitation of this method is the need to balance power to detect interactions with the tendency for models to over-fit the data, given the vast amount of data available. Cross-validation and bootstrapping may help reduce error rates using these models (100). We used recursive partitioning to explore gene by gene interactions in our whole genome data.

1.5 Summary of chapters

In this study, we interrogated naturally occurring genetic variants for association to antidepressant response. The goal of this work is to identify genetic markers that can help guide drug choice or dosing of psychopharmacological therapy with an SSRI. This work was performed using two clinical populations of depressed subjects administered SSRIs: a small (N=96) population taking fluoxetine (Chapters 2 and 3), and a larger (N=1,953) population taking citalopram (Chapters 4, 5, and 6). A flow chart of the projects described in this thesis is shown in Figure 1.1.

In **Chapter 2** of this dissertation, we utilized an LD-based candidate gene approach to investigate likely SSRI pharmacodynamic target genes: serotonin transporter (*SLC6A4*), serotonin 1A, 2A, and 2C receptors (*HTR1A, HTR2A, HTR2C*), tryptophan hydroxylase 1 and 2 (*TPH1* and *TPH2*), and monoamine oxidase A (*MAOA*), for association to fluoxetine response. We genotyped 110 largely non-coding publicly available SNPs and 4 VNTRs across these seven candidate genes. Several SNPs and haplotypes of *SLC6A4, TPH1, TPH2,* and *HTR2A* were nominally associated (p<0.05) with fluoxetine response or response specificity.

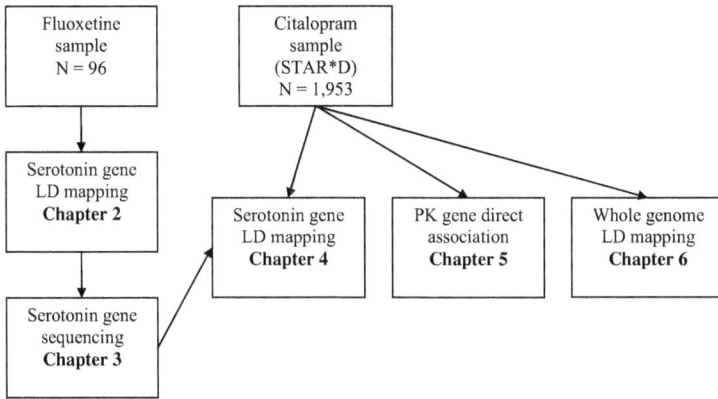

Figure 1.1 Flow chart of work described in this thesis.

Chapter 3 attempts to expand on these results by resequencing the coding regions, intron-exon boundaries and 5' conserved non-coding sequence of these candidate genes in the fluoxetine population. This was performed in order to uncover any potentially functional variants and to capture any additional tagSNPs that were not captured with our genotyping in Chapter 2.

In **Chapter 4**, we utilized the dense marker data (N=188 SNPs) that we had for these pharmacodynamic candidate genes in the fluoxetine population in order to select tagSNPs (N=27) to be genotyped in our larger clinical population taking the SSRI citalopram. No tagSNPs or haplotypes, including the variants that were associated with fluoxetine response in Chapter 1, were significantly associated with citalopram response or response specificity.

Chapter 5 explores the role of pharmacokinetic gene variants in SSRI response. We utilized a direct association approach with known functional variants to investigate the relevant pharmacokinetic genes for citalopram: cytochrome P450 enzymes *CYP3A4*, *CYP3A5*, *CYP2D6* and *CYP2C19*, and P-glycoprotein (*ABCB1*), for association to citalopram response and intolerance. In order to limit Type 1 error we used a two-stage study design. None of the variants that were nominally associated with remission or intolerance in the discovery set were also associated in the validation set. A trend was seen with the *CYP2C19**2 variant and intolerance in the overall sample (p<0.01), however this is not significant given the large number of independent tests performed.

In **Chapter 6**, we make use of a gene-agnostic approach by genotyping approximately 590,000 SNP markers spread across the genome in the discovery set of the citalopram population. The most strongly associated SNPs were then genotyped

19

in the remaining half of the citalopram population, in an effort to validate the initial association.

We attempted to replicate four SNPs that were most highly associated with remission and five SNPs that were most highly associated with intolerance. None of these SNPs replicated their initial association in the validation set, though one SNP in the intolerance phenotype was close (p=0.06). We also attempted to construct multi-SNP decision trees in the discovery set, but again, these models did not replicate in the validation set. However, the analysis presented here of the whole genome data was designed to investigate only the "low hanging fruit", and additional, more comprehensive genotyping of the validation set may yield interesting results. The whole genome work may also identify potential pathways for citalopram's molecular mechanism of action, which is not fully understood.

Chapter 7 summarizes these results and discusses the current challenges facing pharmacogenetics and complex disease association mapping in general, and offers suggestions for future directions.

1.6 References

1.   Kessler RC, Berglund P, Demler O, Jin R, Koretz D, Merikangas KR, Rush AJ, Walters EE, Wang PS. The epidemiology of major depressive disorder: results from the National Comorbidity Survey Replication (NCS-R). *JAMA* 2003; 289(23):3095-3105.

2.   Wong ML, Licinio J. Research and treatment approaches to depression. *Nat Rev Neurosci* 2001; 2(5):343-351.

3.   Hoyert DL, Heron MP, Murphy SL, Kung HC. Deaths: final data for 2003. *Natl Vital Stat Rep* 2006; 54(13):1-120.

4.   Luppa M, Heinrich S, Angermeyer MC, Konig HH, Riedel-Heller SG. Cost-of-illness studies of depression: A systematic review. *J Affect Disord* 2007; 98(1-2):29-43.

5.   Berto P, D'Ilario D, Ruffo P, Di VR, Rizzo F. Depression: cost-of-illness studies in the international literature, a review. *J Ment Health Policy Econ* 2000; 3(1):3-10.

6.   The Global Burden of Disease. Cambridge, Harvard University Press, 1996.

7.   Mueller TI, Leon AC, Keller MB, Solomon DA, Endicott J, Coryell W, Warshaw M, Maser JD. Recurrence after recovery from major depressive disorder during 15 years of observational follow-up. *Am J Psychiarty* 1999; 156(7):1000-1006.

8.   American Psychiatric Association: Diagnostic and Statistical Manual of Mental Disorders, 4th Edition. 1994.

9.   Evans DL, Charney DS, Lewis L, Golden RN, Gorman JM, Krishnan KRR, Nemeroff CB, Bremner JD, Carney RM, Coyne JC. Mood disorders in the medically ill: scientific review and recommendations. *Biol Psychiatry* 2005; 58(3):175-189.

10.   Pincus HA, Pettit AR. The societal costs of chronic major depression. *J Clin Psychiatry* 2001; 62 Suppl 65-9.

11.   Duval F, Lebowitz BD, Macher JP. Treatments in depression. *Dialogues Clin Neurosci* 2006; 8(2):191-206.

12.   Pacher P, Kecskemeti V. Trends in the development of new antidepressants. Is there a light at the end of the tunnel? *Curr Med Chem* 2004; 11(7):925-943.

13.   Stafford RS, MacDonald EA, Finkelstein SN. National patterns of medication treatment for depression, 1987 to 2001. *Prim Care Companion J Clin Psychiatry* 2001; 3(6):232-235.

14.   Stahl SM, Entsuah R, Rudolph RL. Comparative efficacy between venlafaxine and SSRIs: a pooled analysis of patients with depression. *Biol Psychiatry* 2002; 52(12):1166-1174.

15.   Entsuah AR, Huang H, Thase ME. Response and remission rates in different subpopulations with major depressive disorder administered venlafaxine, selective serotonin reuptake inhibitors, or placebo. *J Clin Psychiatry* 2001; 62(11):869-877.

16.   Esposito K, Goodnick P. Predictors of response in depression. *Psychiatr Clin North Am* 2003; 26(2):353-365.

17.   Perlis RH, Iosifescu DV, Renshaw PF. Biological predictors of treatment response in affective illness. *Psychiatr Clin North Am* 2003; 26(2):323-44, vii.

18.   Fergusson D, Doucette S, Glass KC, Shapiro S, Healy D, Hebert P, Hutton B. Association between suicide attempts and selective serotonin reuptake inhibitors: systematic review of randomised controlled trials. *BMJ* 2005; 330(7488):396.

19.   Simon GE, Savarino J, Operskalski B, Wang PS. Suicide risk during antidepressant treatment. *Am J Psychiatry* 2006; 163(1):41-47.

20.   Weber WW: Pharmacogenetics. New York, Oxford University Press, 1997.

21.   Evans WE, Relling MV. Moving towards individualized medicine with pharmacogenomics. *Nature* 2004; 429(6990):464-468.

22.   Ingelman-Sundberg M, Oscarson M, Daly AK, Garte S, Nebert DW. Human

cytochrome P-450 (CYP) genes: a web page for the nomenclature of alleles. *Cancer

Epidemiol Biomarkers Prev* 2001; 10(12):1307-1308.

23.   Weinshilboum R. Inheritance and drug response. *N Engl J Med* 2003;

348(6):529-537.

24.   Drysdale CM, McGraw DW, Stack CB, Stephens JC, Judson RS, Nandabalan

K, Arnold K, Ruano G, Liggett SB. Complex promoter and coding region beta 2-

adrenergic receptor haplotypes alter receptor expression and predict in vivo

responsiveness. *Proc Natl Acad Sci U S A* 2000; 97(19):10483-10488.

25.   Rieder MJ, Reiner AP, Gage BF, Nickerson DA, Eby CS, McLeod HL, Blough

DK, Thummel KE, Veenstra DL, Rettie AE. Effect of VKORC1 haplotypes on

transcriptional regulation and warfarin dose. *N Engl J Med* 2005; 352(22):2285-2293.

26.   Pare CMB, Rees L, Sainsbury MJ. Differentiation of two genetically specific

types of depression by the response to anti-depressants. *Lancet* 1962; 21340-1343.

27.   Pare CMB, Mack JW. Differentiation of two genetically specific types of

depression by the response to antidepressant drugs. *J Med Genet* 1971; 8306-309.

28.   Franchini L, Serretti A, Gasperini M, Smeraldi E. Familial concordance of

fluvoxamine response as a tool for differentiating mood disorder pedigrees. *J

Psychiatr Res* 1998; 32(5):255-259.

29.   O'Reilly RL, Bogue L, Singh SM. Pharmacogenetic response to antidepressants

in a multicase family with affective disorder. *Biol Psychiatry* 1994; 36(7):467-471.

30.   Burke MJ, Preskorn SH. Therapeutic drug monitoring of antidepressants: cost

implications and relevance to clinical practice. *Clin Pharmacokinet* 1999; 37(2):147-

165.

31.   Chen S, Chou WH, Blouin RA, Mao Z, Humphries LL, Meek QC, Neill JR, Martin WL, Hays LR, Wedlund PJ. The cytochrome P450 2D6 (CYP2D6) enzyme polymorphism: screening costs and influence on clinical outcomes in psychiatry. *Clin Pharmacol Ther* 1996; 60(5):522-534.

32.   Kvist EE, Al Shurbaji A, Dahl ML, Nordin C, Alvan G, Stahle L. Quantitative pharmacogenetics of nortriptyline: a novel approach. *Clin Pharmacokinet* 2001; 40(11):869-877.

33.   Kirchheiner J, Brosen K, Dahl ML, Gram LF, Kasper S, Roots I, Sjoqvist F, Spina E, Brockmoller J. CYP2D6 and CYP2C19 genotype-based dose recommendations for antidepressants: a first step towards subpopulation-specific dosages. *Acta Psychiatr Scand* 2001; 104(3):173-192.

34.   Mrazek DA, Smoller JW, de LJ. Incorporating pharmacogenetics into clinical practice: Reality of a new tool in psychiatry. *CNS Spectr* 2006; 11(3 Suppl 3):1-13.

35.   de Leon J, Susce MT, Murray-Carmichael E. The AmpliChip CYP450 genotyping test: Integrating a new clinical tool. *Mol Diagn Ther* 2006; 10(3):135-151.

36.   Lerer B, Macciardi F. Pharmacogenetics of antidepressant and mood-stabilizing drugs: a review of candidate-gene studies and future research directions. *Int J Neuropsychopharmacol* 2002; 5(3):255-275.

37.   Yu YWY, Tsai SJ, Liou YJ, Hong CJ, Chen TJ. Association study of two serotonin 1A receptor gene polymorphisms and fluoxetine treatment response in Chinese major depressive disorders. *Eur Neuropsychopharmacol* 2006; 16(7):498-503.

38.   Cusin C, Serretti A, Zanardi R, Lattuada E, Rossini D, Lilli R, Lorenzi C, Smeraldi E. Influence of monoamine oxidase A and serotonin receptor 2A

polymorphisms in SSRI antidepressant activity. *Int J Neuropsychopharmacol* 2002; 5(1):27-35.

39.   Yoshida K, Naito S, Takahashi H, Sato K, Ito K, Kamata M, Higuchi H, Shimizu T, Itoh K, Inoue K, Tezuka T, Suzuki T, Ohkubo T, Sugawara K, Otani K. Monoamine oxidase: A gene polymorphism, tryptophan hydroxylase gene polymorphism and antidepressant response to fluvoxamine in Japanese patients with major depressive disorder. *Prog Neuropsychopharmacol Biol Psychiatry* 2002; 26(7-8):1279-1283.

40.   Serretti A, Zanardi R, Rossini D, Cusin C, Lilli R, Smeraldi E. Influence of tryptophan hydroxylase and serotonin transporter genes on fluvoxamine antidepressant activity. *Mol Psychiatry* 2001; 6(5):586-592.

41.   Serretti A, Zanardi R, Cusin C, Rossini D, Lorenzi C, Smeraldi E. Tryptophan hydroxylase gene associated with paroxetine antidepressant activity. *Eur Neuropsychopharmacol* 2001; 11(5):375-380.

42.   Smeraldi E, Zanardi R, Benedetti F, Di Bella D, Perez J, Catalano M. Polymorphism within the promoter of the serotonin transporter gene and antidepressant efficacy of fluvoxamine. *Mol Psychiatry* 1998; 3(6):508-511.

43.   Zanardi R, Benedetti F, Di Bella D, Catalano M, Smeraldi E. Efficacy of paroxetine in depression is influenced by a functional polymorphism within the promoter of the serotonin transporter gene. *J Clin Psychopharmacol* 2000; 20(1):105-107.

44.   Zanardi R, Serretti A, Rossini D, Franchini L, Cusin C, Lattuada E, Dotoli D, Smeraldi E. Factors affecting fluvoxamine antidepressant activity: influence of pindolol and 5-HTTLPR in delusional and nondelusional depression. *Biol Psychiatry* 2001; 50(5):323-330.

45.   Kim DK, Lim SW, Lee S, Sohn SE, Kim S, Hahn CG, Carroll BJ. Serotonin transporter gene polymorphism and antidepressant response. *NeuroReport* 2000; 11(1):215-219.

46.   Pollock BG, Ferrell RE, Mulsant BH, Mazumdar S, Miller M, Sweet RA, Davis S, Kirshner MA, Houck PR, Stack JA, Reynolds CF, Kupfer DJ. Allelic variation in the serotonin transporter promoter affects onset of paroxetine treatment response in late-life depression. *Neuropsychopharmacology* 2000; 23(5):587-590.

47.   Arias B, Catalan R, Gasto C, Gutierrez B, Fananas L. 5-HTTLPR polymorphism of the serotonin transporter gene predicts non-remission in major depression patients treated with citalopram in a 12-weeks follow up study. *J Clin Psychopharmacol* 2003; 23(6):563-567.

48.   Lesch K-P, Bengel D, Heils A, Sabol SZ, Greenberg BD, Petri S, Benjamin J, Müller CR, Hamer DH, Murphy DL. Association of anxiety-related traits with a polymorphism in the serotonin transporter gene regulatory region. *Science* 1996; 274(5292):1527-1531.

49.   Zill P, Baghai TC, Zwanzger P, Schule C, Minov C, Riedel M, Neumeier K, Rupprecht R, Bondy B. Evidence for an association between a G-protein beta3-gene variant with depression and response to antidepressant treatment. *NeuroReport* 2000; 11(9):1893-1897.

50.   Lee HJ, Cha JH, Ham BJ, Han CS, Kim YK, Lee SH, Ryu SH, Kang RH, Choi MJ, Lee MS. Association between a G-protein beta3 subunit gene polymorphism and the symptomatology and treatment responses of major depressive disorders. *Pharmacogenomics J* 2004; 4(1):29-33.

51.   Baghai TC, Schule C, Zwanzger P, Minov C, Schwarz MJ, de Jonge S, Rupprecht R, Bondy B. Possible influence of the insertion/deletion polymorphism in

the angiotensin I-converting enzyme gene on therapeutic outcome in affective

disorders. *Mol Psychiatry* 2001; 6(3):258-259.

52. Binder EB, Salyakina D, Lichtner P, Wochnik GM, Ising M, Putz B, Papiol S,

Seaman S, Lucae S, Kohli MA, Nickel T, Kunzel HE, Fuchs B, Majer M, Pfennig A,

Kern N, Brunner J, Modell S, Baghai T, Deiml T, Zill P, Bondy B, Rupprecht R,

Messer T, Kohnlein O, Dabitz H, Bruckl T, Muller N, Pfister H, Lieb R, Mueller JC,

Lohmussaar E, Strom TM, Bettecken T, Meitinger T, Uhr M, Rein T, Holsboer F,

Muller-Myhsok B. Polymorphisms in FKBP5 are associated with increased

recurrence of depressive episodes and rapid response to antidepressant treatment. *Nat

Genet* 2004; 36(12):1319-1325.

53. Perlis RH, Mischoulon D, Smoller JW, Wan YJY, Lamon-Fava S, Lin KM,

Rosenbaum JF, Fava M. Serotonin transporter polymorphisms and adverse effects

with fluoxetine treatment. *Biol Psychiatry* 2003; 54(9):879-883.

54. Murphy GM, Jr., Kremer C, Rodrigues HE, Schatzberg AF. Pharmacogenetics

of antidepressant medication intolerance. *Am J Psychiatry* 2003; 160(10):1830-1835.

55. Grasmader K, Verwohlt PL, Rietschel M, Dragicevic A, Muller M, Hiemke C,

Freymann N, Zobel A, Maier W, Rao ML. Impact of polymorphisms of cytochrome-

P450 isoenzymes 2C9, 2C19 and 2D6 on plasma concentrations and clinical effects of

antidepressants in a naturalistic clinical setting. *Eur J Clin Pharmacol* 2004;

60(5):329-336.

56. Yin OQ, Wing YK, Cheung Y, Wang ZJ, Lam SL, Chiu HF, Chow MS.

Phenotype-genotype relationship and clinical effects of citalopram in Chinese

patients. *J Clin Psychopharmacol* 2006; 26(4):367-372.

57. Suzuki Y, Sawamura K, Someya T. Polymorphisms in the 5-hydroxytryptamine

2A receptor and cytochrome P4502D6 genes synergistically predict fluvoxamine-induced side effects in Japanese depressed patients. *Neuropsychopharmacology* 2006; 31(4):825-831.

58.   Lander ES, Linton LM, Birren B, Nusbaum C, Zody MC, Baldwin J, Devon K, Dewar K, Doyle M, FitzHugh W, Funke R, Gage D, Harris K, Heaford A, Howland J, Kann L, Lehoczky J, LeVine R, McEwan P, McKernan K, Meldrim J, Mesirov JP, Miranda C, Morris W, Naylor J, Raymond C, Rosetti M, Santos R, Sheridan A, Sougnez C, Stange-Thomann N, Stojanovic N, Subramanian A, Wyman D, Rogers J, Sulston J, Ainscough R, Beck S, Bentley D, Burton J, Clee C, Carter N, Coulson A, Deadman R, Deloukas P, Dunham A, Dunham I, Durbin R, French L, Grafham D, Gregory S, Hubbard T, Humphray S, Hunt A, Jones M, Lloyd C, McMurray A, Matthews L, Mercer S, Milne S, Mullikin JC, Mungall A, Plumb R, Ross M, Shownkeen R, Sims S, Waterston RH, Wilson RK, Hillier LW, McPherson JD, Marra MA, Mardis ER, Fulton LA, Chinwalla AT, Pepin KH, Gish WR, Chissoe SL, Wendl MC, Delehaunty KD, Miner TL, Delehaunty A, Kramer JB, Cook LL, Fulton RS, Johnson DL, Minx PJ, Clifton SW, Hawkins T, Branscomb E, Predki P, Richardson P, Wenning S, Slezak T, Doggett N, Cheng JF, Olsen A, Lucas S, Elkin C, Uberbacher E, Frazier M, Gibbs RA, Muzny DM, Scherer SE, Bouck JB, Sodergren EJ, Worley KC, Rives CM, Gorrell JH, Metzker ML, Naylor SL, Kucherlapati RS, Nelson DL, Weinstock GM, Sakaki Y, Fujiyama A, Hattori M, Yada T, Toyoda A, Itoh T, Kawagoe C, Watanabe H, Totoki Y, Taylor T, Weissenbach J, Heilig R, Saurin W, Artiguenave F, Brottier P, Bruls T, Pelletier E, Robert C, Wincker P, Smith DR, Doucette-Stamm L, Rubenfield M, Weinstock K, Lee HM, Dubois J, Rosenthal A, Platzer M, Nyakatura G, Taudien S, Rump A, Yang H, Yu J, Wang J, Huang G, Gu J, Hood L, Rowen L, Madan A, Qin S, Davis RW, Federspiel NA, Abola AP, Proctor MJ, Myers RM, Schmutz J, Dickson M, Grimwood J, Cox DR, Olson MV,

Kaul R, Raymond C, Shimizu N, Kawasaki K, Minoshima S, Evans GA, Athanasiou

M, Schultz R, Roe BA, Chen F, Pan H, Ramser J, Lehrach H, Reinhardt R,

McCombie WR, de la BM, Dedhia N, Blocker H, Hornischer K, Nordsiek G,

Agarwala R, Aravind L, Bailey JA, Bateman A, Batzoglou S, Birney E, Bork P,

Brown DG, Burge CB, Cerutti L, Chen HC, Church D, Clamp M, Copley RR, Doerks

T, Eddy SR, Eichler EE, Furey TS, Galagan J, Gilbert JG, Harmon C, Hayashizaki Y,

Haussler D, Hermjakob H, Hokamp K, Jang W, Johnson LS, Jones TA, Kasif S,

Kaspryzk A, Kennedy S, Kent WJ, Kitts P, Koonin EV, Korf I, Kulp D, Lancet D,

Lowe TM, McLysaght A, Mikkelsen T, Moran JV, Mulder N, Pollara VJ, Ponting CP,

Schuler G, Schultz J, Slater G, Smit AF, Stupka E, Szustakowski J, Thierry-Mieg D,

Thierry-Mieg J, Wagner L, Wallis J, Wheeler R, Williams A, Wolf YI, Wolfe KH,

Yang SP, Yeh RF, Collins F, Guyer MS, Peterson J, Felsenfeld A, Wetterstrand KA,

Patrinos A, Morgan MJ, Szustakowki J, de Jong P, Catanese JJ, Osoegawa K, Shizuya

H, Choi S. Initial sequencing and analysis of the human genome. *Nature* 2001;

409(6822):860-921.

59.   Venter JC, Adams MD, Myers EW, Li PW, Mural RJ, Sutton GG, Smith HO,

Yandell M, Evans CA, Holt RA, Gocayne JD, Amanatides P, Ballew RM, Huson DH,

Wortman JR, Zhang Q, Kodira CD, Zheng XH, Chen L, Skupski M, Subramanian G,

Thomas PD, Zhang J, Gabor Miklos GL, Nelson C, Broder S, Clark AG, Nadeau J,

McKusick VA, Zinder N, Levine AJ, Roberts RJ, Simon M, Slayman C, Hunkapiller

M, Bolanos R, Delcher A, Dew I, Fasulo D, Flanigan M, Florea L, Halpern A,

Hannenhalli S, Kravitz S, Levy S, Mobarry C, Reinert K, Remington K, Abu-

Threideh J, Beasley E, Biddick K, Bonazzi V, Brandon R, Cargill M,

Chandramouliswaran I, Charlab R, Chaturvedi K, Deng Z, Di F, V, Dunn P, Eilbeck

K, Evangelista C, Gabrielian AE, Gan W, Ge W, Gong F, Gu Z, Guan P, Heiman TJ,

Higgins ME, Ji RR, Ke Z, Ketchum KA, Lai Z, Lei Y, Li Z, Li J, Liang Y, Lin X, Lu F, Merkulov GV, Milshina N, Moore HM, Naik AK, Narayan VA, Neelam B, Nusskern D, Rusch DB, Salzberg S, Shao W, Shue B, Sun J, Wang Z, Wang A, Wang X, Wang J, Wei M, Wides R, Xiao C, Yan C, Yao A, Ye J, Zhan M, Zhang W, Zhang H, Zhao Q, Zheng L, Zhong F, Zhong W, Zhu S, Zhao S, Gilbert D, Baumhueter S, Spier G, Carter C, Cravchik A, Woodage T, Ali F, An H, Awe A, Baldwin D, Baden H, Barnstead M, Barrow I, Beeson K, Busam D, Carver A, Center A, Cheng ML, Curry L, Danaher S, Davenport L, Desilets R, Dietz S, Dodson K, Doup L, Ferriera S, Garg N, Gluecksmann A, Hart B, Haynes J, Haynes C, Heiner C, Hladun S, Hostin D, Houck J, Howland T, Ibegwam C, Johnson J, Kalush F, Kline L, Koduru S, Love A, Mann F, May D, McCawley S, McIntosh T, McMullen I, Moy M, Moy L, Murphy B, Nelson K, Pfannkoch C, Pratts E, Puri V, Qureshi H, Reardon M, Rodriguez R, Rogers YH, Romblad D, Ruhfel B, Scott R, Sitter C, Smallwood M, Stewart E, Strong R, Suh E, Thomas R, Tint NN, Tse S, Vech C, Wang G, Wetter J, Williams S, Williams M, Windsor S, Winn-Deen E, Wolfe K, Zaveri J, Zaveri K, Abril JF, Guigo R, Campbell MJ, Sjolander KV, Karlak B, Kejariwal A, Mi H, Lazareva B, Hatton T, Narechania A, Diemer K, Muruganujan A, Guo N, Sato S, Bafna V, Istrail S, Lippert R, Schwartz R, Walenz B, Yooseph S, Allen D, Basu A, Baxendale J, Blick L, Caminha M, Carnes-Stine J, Caulk P, Chiang YH, Coyne M, Dahlke C, Mays A, Dombroski M, Donnelly M, Ely D, Esparham S, Fosler C, Gire H, Glanowski S, Glasser K, Glodek A, Gorokhov M, Graham K, Gropman B, Harris M, Heil J, Henderson S, Hoover J, Jennings D, Jordan C, Jordan J, Kasha J, Kagan L, Kraft C, Levitsky A, Lewis M, Liu X, Lopez J, Ma D, Majoros W, McDaniel J, Murphy S, Newman M, Nguyen T, Nguyen N, Nodell M. The sequence of the human genome. *Science* 2001; 291(5507):1304-1351.

60. Kwok PY. Methods for genotyping single nucleotide polymorphisms. *Annu Rev Genomics Hum Genet* 2001; 2235-258.

61. Dermitzakis ET, Reymond A, Scamuffa N, Ucla C, Kirkness E, Rossier C, Antonarakis SE. Evolutionary discrimination of mammalian conserved non-genic sequences (CNGs). *Science* 2003; 302(5647):1033-1035.

62. Wang QF, Prabhakar S, Chanan S, Cheng JF, Boffelli D, Rubin EM. Detection of weakly conserved ancestral mammalian regulatory sequences by primate comparisons. *Genome Biol* 2007; advanced online publication.

63. Risch N, Merikangas K. The future of genetic studies of complex human diseases. *Science* 1996; 273(5281):1516-1517.

64. Ott J, Hoh J. Statistical approaches to gene mapping. *Am J Hum Genet* 2000; 67(2):289-294.

65. Cardon LR, Bell JI. Association study designs for complex diseases. *Nat Rev Genet* 2001; 2(2):91-99.

66. Risch N, Teng J. The relative power of family-based and case-control designs for linkage disequilibrium studies of complex human diseases. *Genome Res* 1998; 8(12):1273-1288.

67. Zondervan KT, Cardon LR. The complex interplay among factors that influence allelic association. *Nat Rev Genet* 2004; 5(2):89-100.

68. Collins FS, Guyer MS, Charkravarti A. Variations on a theme: cataloging human DNA sequence variation. *Science* 1997; 278(5343):1580-1581.

69. Reich DE, Lander ES. On the allelic spectrum of human disease. *Trends in Genetics* 2001; 17(9):502-510.

70. Clark AG. The role of haplotypes in candidate gene studies. *Genet Epidemiol* 2004; 27(4):321-333.

71.   Newton-Cheh C, Hirschhorn JN. Genetic association studies of complex traits: design and analysis issues. *Mutat Res* 2005; 573(1-2):54-69.

72.   Weiss KM, Terwilliger JD. How many diseases does it take to map a gene with SNPs? *Nat Genet* 2000; 26(2):151-157.

73.   Pritchard JK. Are rare variants responsible for susceptibility to complex diseases? *Am J Hum Genet* 2001; 69(1):124-137.

74.   Wen G, Mahata SK, Cadman P, Mahata M, Ghosh S, Mahapatra NR, Rao F, Stridsberg M, Smith DW, Mahboubi P, Schork NJ, O'Connor DT, Hamilton BA. Both rare and common polymorphisms contribute functional variation at CHGA, a regulator of catecholamine physiology. *Am J Hum Genet* 2004; 74(2):197-207.

75.   Maraganore DM, de Andrade M, Lesnick TG, Strain KJ, Farrer MJ, Rocca WA, Pant PVK, Frazer KA, Cox DR, Ballinger DG. High-resolution whole-genome association study of Parkinson disease. *Am J Hum Genet* 2005; 77(5):685-693.

76.   Klein RJ, Zeiss C, Chew EY, Tsai JY, Sackler RS, Haynes C, Henning AK, SanGiovanni JP, Mane SM, Mayne ST, Bracken MB, Ferris FL, Ott J, Barnstable C, Hoh J. Complement Factor H polymorphism in age-related macular degeneration. *Science* 2005; 308(5720):385-9.

77.   Lawrence RW, Evans DM, Cardon LR. Prospects and pitfalls in whole genome association studies. *Philos Trans R Soc Lond B Biol Sci* 2005; 360(1460):1589-1595.

78.   Herbert A, Gerry NP, McQueen MB, Heid IM, Pfeufer A, Illig T, Wichmann HE, Meitinger T, Hunter D, Hu FB, Colditz G, Hinney A, Hebebrand J, Koberwitz K, Zhu X, Cooper R, Ardlie K, Lyon H, Hirschhorn JN, Laird NM, Lenburg ME, Lange C, Christman MF. A common genetic variant is associated with adult and childhood obesity. *Science* 2006; 312(5771):279-283.

79.   Quitkin FM, Rabkin JD, Markowitz JM, Stewart JW, McGrath, PJ, Harrison W. Use of pattern analysis to identify true drug response. A replication. *Arch Gen Psychiatry* 1987; 44(3):259-264.

80.   McGrath PJ, Stewart JW, Petkova E, Quitkin FM, Amsterdam JD, Fawcett J, Reimherr FW, Rosenbaum JF, Beasley CM, Jr. Predictors of relapse during fluoxetine continuation or maintenance treatment of major depression. *J Clin Psychiatry* 2000; 61(7):518-524.

81.   McGrath PJ, Stewart JW, Quitkin FM, Chen Y, Alpert JE, Nierenberg AA, Fava M, Cheng J, Petkova E. Predictors of relapse in a prospective study of fluoxetine treatment of major depression. *Am J Psychiatry* 2006; 163(9):1542-1548.

82.   Carlson CS, Eberle MA, Rieder MJ, Yi Q, Kruglyak L, Nickerson DA. Selecting a maximally informative set of single-nucleotide polymorphisms for association analyses using linkage disequilibrium. *Am J Hum Genet* 2004; 74(1):106-120.

83.   Ke X, Cardon LR. Efficient selective screening of haplotype tag SNPs. *Bioinformatics* 2003; 19(2):287-288.

84.   Stram DO, Haiman CA, Hirschhorn JN, Altshuler D, Kolonel LN, Henderson BE, Pike MC. Choosing haplotype-tagging SNPS based on unphased genotype data using a preliminary sample of unrelated subjects with an example from the Multiethnic Cohort Study. *Hum Hered* 2003; 55(1):27-36.

85.   Weale ME, Depondt C, Macdonald SJ, Smith A, Lai PS, Shorvon SD, Wood NW, Goldstein DB. Selection and evaluation of tagging SNPs in the neuronal-sodium-channel gene SCN1A: implications for linkage-disequilibrium gene mapping. *Am J Hum Genet* 2003; 73(3):551-565.

86. Devlin B, Roeder K, Wasserman L. Analysis of multilocus models of association. *Genet Epidemiol* 2003; 25(1):36-47.

87. Dudbridge F, Koeleman BP. Efficient computation of significance levels for multiple associations in large studies of correlated data, including genomewide association studies. *Am J Hum Genet* 2004; 75(3):424-435.

88. Storey JD, Tibshirani R. Statistical significance for genomewide studies. *Proc Natl Acad Sci U S A* 2003; 100(16):9440-9445.

89. Wang H, Thomas DC, Pe'er I, Stram DO. Optimal two-stage genotyping designs for genome-wide association scans. *Genet Epidemiol* 2006; 30(4):356-368.

90. Skol AD, Scott LJ, Abecasis GR, Boehnke M. Joint analysis is more efficient than replication-based analysis for two-stage genome-wide association studies. *Nat Genet* 2006; 38(2):209-213.

91. Laird NM, Lange C. Family-based designs in the age of large-scale gene-association studies. *Nat Rev Genet* 2006; 7(5):385-394.

92. Cardon LR, Palmer LJ. Population stratification and spurious allelic association. *Lancet* 2003; 361(9357):598-604.

93. Tang H, Quertermous T, Rodriguez B, Kardia SL, Zhu X, Brown A, Pankow JS, Province MA, Hunt SC, Boerwinkle E, Schork NJ, Risch NJ. Genetic structure, self-identified race/ethnicity, and confounding in case-control association studies. *Am J Hum Genet* 2005; 76(2):268-275.

94. Shriver MD, Mei R, Parra EJ, Sonpar V, Halder I, Tishkoff SA, Schurr TG, Zhadanov SI, Osipova LP, Brutsaert TD, Friedlaender J, Jorde LB, Watkins WS, Bamshad MJ, Gutierrez G, Loi H, Matsuzaki H, Kittles RA, Argyropoulos G, Fernandez JR, Akey JM, Jones KW. Large-scale SNP analysis reveals clustered and continuous patterns of human genetic variation. *Hum Genomics* 2005; 2(2):81-89.

95. Devlin B, Roeder K, Wasserman L. Genomic control, a new approach to genetic-based association studies. *Theor Popul Biol* 2001; 60(3):155-166.

96. Pritchard JK, Rosenberg NA. Use of unlinked genetic markers to detect population stratification in association studies. *Am J Hum Genet* 1999; 65(1):220-228.

97. Falush D, Stephens M, Pritchard JK. Inference of population structure using multilocus genotype data: linked loci and correlated allele frequencies. *Genetics* 2003; 164(4):1567-1587.

98. Heidema AG, Boer JM, Nagelkerke N, Mariman EC, van der AD, Feskens EJ. The challenge for genetic epidemiologists: how to analyze large numbers of SNPs in relation to complex diseases. *BMC Genet* 2006; Apr 21:7-23.

99. Young SS, Ge N. Recursive partitioning analysis of complex disease pharmacogenetic studies: I. Motivation and overview. *Pharmacogenomics* 2005; 6(1):65-75.

100. Zaykin DV, Young SS. Large recursive partitioning analysis of complex disease pharmacogenetic studies: II. Statistical considerations. *Pharmacogenomics* 2005; 6(1):77-89.

CHAPTER 2

LINKAGE DISEQUILIBRIUM MAPPING OF VARIANTS IN

PHARMACODYNAMIC CANDIDATE GENES FOR ASSOCIATION WITH

RESPONSE TO FLUOXETINE[*]

2.1 Introduction

Major depression has one of the highest lifetime incidence rates among

psychiatric disorders (1;2). Thus, antidepressant medications are among the most

commonly prescribed pharmacological agents. However, despite recent advances in

antidepressant pharmacotherapy, patient response rates can still be as low as 60% for

the first drug administered (3). Inter-individual variation in antidepressant efficacy is

thought to be at least partly under genetic control (4-6). Selective serotonin reuptake

inhibitors (SSRIs), commonly prescribed medications, are believed to exert their

antidepressant effect through inhibiting the serotonin transporter, which terminates

serotonin (5-HT) transmission. A number of studies have tested the association

between DNA variations in the serotonin transporter and response to various SSRI's

(4). The majority of these studies rely on assaying a common insertion/deletion

polymorphism in the *SLC6A4* promoter that alters in vitro transcription of the gene

(7). This 43 base pair insertion/deletion primarily comes in long ("l") and short ("s")

forms, with the long form being more transcriptionally active *in vitro*. In Caucasian

subjects taking SSRIs, the presence of the long allele has been associated with

response in multiple studies (8),

---

[*] This chapter has been published previously: Peters E.J., Slager S.L., McGrath P.J., Knowles J.A., Hamilton S.P. "Investigation serotonin-related genes in antidepressant response." *Molecular Psychiatry* 2004; 9(9): 879-889. Reprinted with permission

while in a Korean population, the short allele has been associated with a more favorable response (9). In a second Korean population, the long allele was associated with a better response (10). The reason for this discrepancy has not been addressed, but is likely to involve the unique population histories of the *SLC6A4* locus between the European/U.S. subjects and the Asian subjects (for detailed summary see (11)). Furthermore, even in positive studies, this polymorphism does not explain all of the variance seen in response suggesting the involvement of other variants within other genes or environmental factors.

As serotonin appears to play an important role in depression, we first chose to pursue an analysis of a group of genes in the serotonin pathway. These genes are involved with the synthesis, signal transduction, transport, and catabolism of serotonin. Tryptophan hydroxylase (TPH1) catalyzes the rate-limiting step in the biosynthesis of 5-HT. Recently, Walther *et al.* described a second isoform of tryptophan hydroxylase (TPH2), which was shown to be the major form expressed in the brain, with TPH1 being expressed mainly in the periphery (12), although central TPH1 function in early development appears critical (13). Serotonin receptors 1A (HTR1A), 2A (HTR2A), and 2C (HTR2C) are involved in the neurotransmission of 5-HT. The serotonin transporter (*SLC6A4*), is involved with clearing the synapse of 5-HT. Finally, monoamine oxidase A (MAOA) is one of the main enzymes involved in the degradation of 5-HT. Monoamine oxidase inhibitors have been used for decades to treat Major Depressive Disorder. SSRIs have antagonistic properties at serotonin receptors, while the functional effect of SSRIs, increased synaptic 5-HT, has an indirect effect on HTR1A, HTR2A, and HTR2C function (14-16). SSRIs can modulate the expression of tryptophan hydroxylase mRNA, and inhibition of tryptophan hydroxylase activity has dramatic effects on brain serotonin levels (17-19).

A number of studies have individually investigated the role of several of these genes in antidepressant response (20-23).

Given the small number of reports at the time the work described in this chapter was performed, as well as biological data implicating their role in serotonergic function, we investigated the association between treatment response to fluoxetine and a large number of publicly available SNPs (N=110) in *TPH1*, *TPH2*, *HTR1A*, *HTR2A*, *HTR2C*, *SLC6A4*, and *MAOA*. We used a well-phenotyped population of persons with unipolar major depression and carried out an analysis of association between these variants and response to fluoxetine. We attempted to limit phenotypic heterogeneity through use of response pattern analysis that classifies patients as non-responders, specific responders, or placebo responders to fluoxetine (24). We also utilized both single SNPs as well as haplotypes for detecting an association to SSRI response and a genomic control technique to correct for possible population stratification.

2.2 Methods

2.2.1 Fluoxetine study population. The study population consisted of 96 research subjects enrolled in an ongoing NIMH-funded protocol (Patrick J. McGrath, Columbia University, principal investigator) to assess relapse following fluoxetine discontinuation in depressed subjects who had responded to fluoxetine. Inclusion in that clinical trial required subjects to be in a current episode of Major Depression, to be aged 18-65 years, and to give informed consent to be randomized to either fluoxetine continuation or to placebo substitution should they respond to acute treatment (24;25). There was no depression severity threshold for inclusion. The Structured Clinical Interview for DSM-IV Axis I Disorders - Patient Edition (SCID-

I/P) was used to establish all psychiatric diagnoses (26). Subjects with any history of psychosis, mania, organic mental syndrome, a history of substance abuse or dependence active within the previous six months, with the exception of nicotine dependence, current bulimia nervosa, or unstable physical illnesses were excluded. Other Axis I co-morbid disorders were not exclusionary. Medications known to cause or exacerbate depression, such as beta-blockers or corticosteroids, or to have significant anitidepressant or anxiolytic properties, were exclusionary. Study subjects were included if they took occasional hypnotic medication of a non-benzodiazepine type, oral contraceptives which were not temporally associated with onset or exacerbation of depression, or thyroid hormone replacement which was at a constant and effective dose for three months prior to study. Concomitant medications such as diuretics and antihypertensives were permitted. Only data from the initial 12 week trial were used in these analyses as the number of subjects was considered to be inadequate to use follow-up data where subjects were randomized to fluoxetine or placebo and either maintained their response or relapsed (25).

Patients were categorized as non-responders, specific pattern responders, or placebo-pattern responders by pattern analysis after 12 weeks of open-label fluoxetine treatment (24). Fluoxetine daily dosage was 10 mg for one week, 20 mg daily for three weeks, 40 mg for four weeks, and 60 mg for the remaining four weeks. Dosage increments were made only in those tolerating the medication well and insufficiently responsive to 40 mg. Response in any week was judged by the use of the Clinical Global Impression Improvement score where a score of "much improved" or "very much improved" was required for response. This criterion was applied with the definition that "much improved" characterized someone that the clinician believed was sufficiently improved that no change in treatment was warranted. This usually corresponded to a decrement of between 50 and 75% in baseline depression ratings on the Hamilton Depression Scale, the traditional measure of antidepressant efficacy. Subjects responding at week 12 whose response began after the second week and were sustained until week 12 were considered "specific-pattern" responders; subjects whose response began in weeks one or two but whose response was not sustained for all subsequent weeks until week 12 were considered "placebo-pattern" or "non-specific" responders. In short, pattern analysis draws on the observation that a specific response to medication is associated with a delayed response to active medication that is persistent once achieved, while a non-specific response has an earlier onset of response and/or lack of persistence in improvement after onset. This is based on the observation, replicated in several independent samples, that "placebo" or "non-specific" patterns are found equally among patients on active drug and on placebo, while only specific patterns are significantly more common on active medication (25;27). While pattern analysis clearly does not perfectly characterize placebo and active medication response (28), it is an attempt to deal with the problem that approximately half of all subjects (one quarter in this study) who respond to medication treatment are having a placebo response (29). Informed consent was obtained from each research participant, as was IRB approval from the New York State Psychiatric Institute and the University of California at San Francisco. In this group, the average age was 37.1 ± 11.6 years, and the male/female ratio was 47 to 49. There were 77 (80%) responders and 19 (20%) non-responders to a 12-week trial of fluoxetine. The subjects were 78% Caucasian, 6% African-American, 7% Hispanic, 5% Asian, and 3% other. There were no significant differences in ethnicity (by exact test, $p=0.07$) or age (by t-test, $p=0.19$) between responders and non-responders.

Using a clinical pattern analysis paradigm, 20 of the 77 responders (26%) were determined to be "non-specific" responders to fluoxetine (Figure 2.1).

Four chimpanzee (*Pan troglodytes*) and one bonobo (*Pan paniscus*) genomic DNA samples were obtained from the Coriell Institute for use in determining the ancestral allele at candidate SNPs (Coriell Institute for Medical Research, Camden, NJ) (30).

2.2.2 SSRI pharmacodynamic gene SNP genotyping. Patient genomic DNA was extracted from whole blood using a Puregene genomic DNA purification kit (Gentra Systems, Minneapolis, MN). DNA was quantified using a ND-1000 spectrophotometer (NanoDrop Technologies, Rockland, DE).

A total of 165 SNPs were identified from publicly available databases or the literature and were chosen with an unbiased approach in an effort to distribute them evenly across the seven candidate genes (Figure 2.2). These SNPs, very few of which were previously validated, represented the best available at the time these experiments were carried out. SNPs in the 5' and 3' region flanking the gene were also included in this study. One hundred ten of the 165 were used for genotyping, as 32 were monomorphic in our population and an adequate SNP genotyping assay could not be developed for the final 23. Of the 110 SNPs used in this study, 66 were intronic, 10 were exonic (4 non-synonymous and 6 synonymous changes), and 34 were located in the 5' and 3' flanking regions. Fluorescence polarization detection of template-directed dye-terminator incorporation (FP-TDI) was used to genotype SNPs, as described elsewhere (31;32). Briefly, the first step involves polymerase chain reactions (PCR) of 5 microliters (µl) containing 200 nM of the forward and reverse primers (Table 2.1), 20 ng genomic DNA template, 50 µM dNTPs (Roche, Indianapolis, IN), 1M anhydrous betaine (Acros Organics, Geel, Belgium), 50 mM

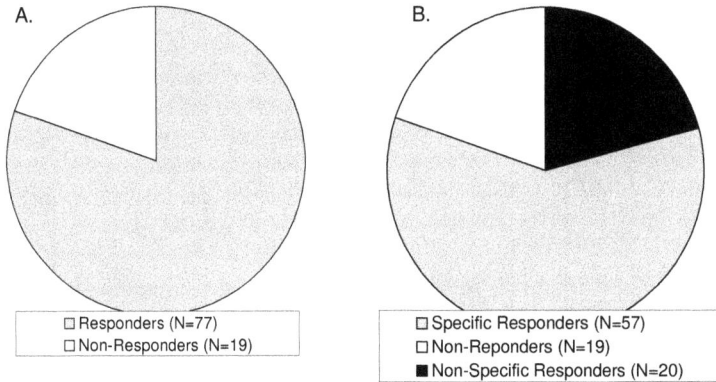

A.

☐ Responders (N=77)
☐ Non-Responders (N=19)

B.

☐ Specific Responders (N=57)
☐ Non-Reponders (N=19)
■ Non-Specific Responders (N=20)

Figure 2.1. Phenotype classifications in the fluoxetine sample set. A.) Breakdown of sample by primary phenotype comparison of categorical responders versus non-responders. B.) Additional sub-classification of sample set based on specific and non-specific response.

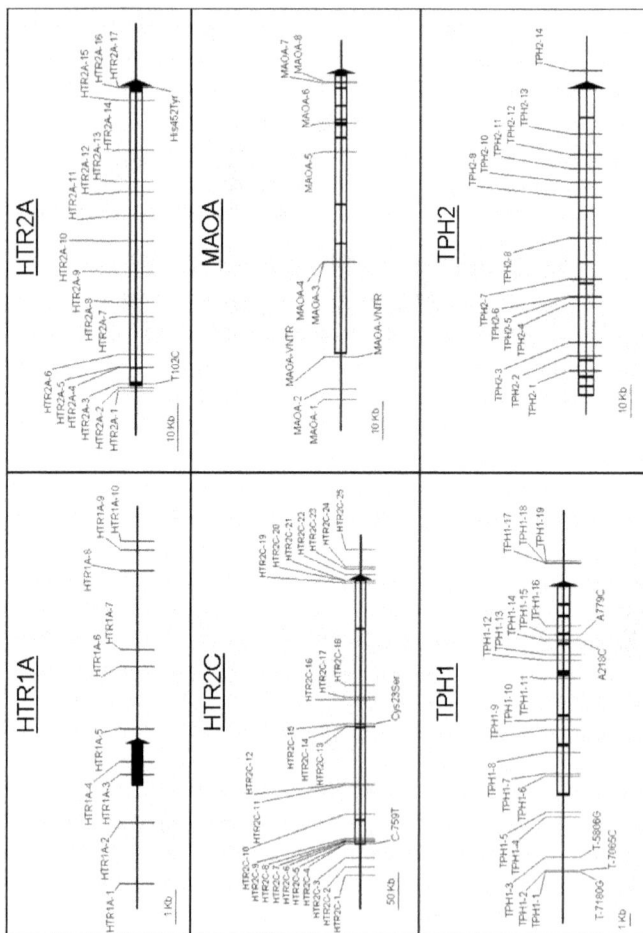

Figure 2.2. Pharmacodynamic candidate gene schematics.

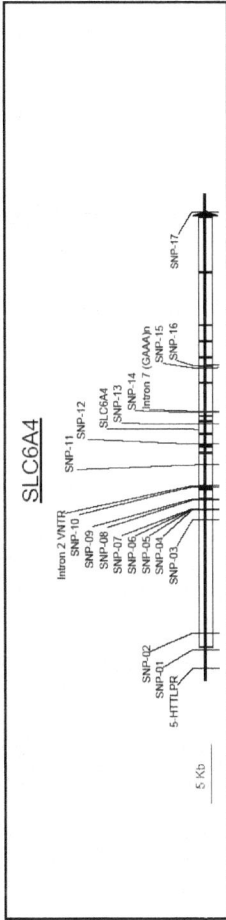

Figure 2.2 (continued). Pharmacodynamic candidate gene schematics. Schematic diagrams of the seven serotonergic genes studied. Genes are showing in the 5' to 3' direction with solid boxes representing exons. SNPs assayed are shown as vertical lines with nomenclature used in this paper given above the gene and any alternative nomenclature given below the gene.

KCl, 20mM Tris-HCl (pH 8.4), 2.5 mM $MgCl_2$, and 0.25 units Platinum Taq DNA polymerase (Invitrogen, Carlsbad, CA). All primers and TDI probes were designed using Primer3 software and were manufactured by Invitrogen (Carlsbad, CA) (33). Samples were cycled using a touchdown protocol at 94°C for 3 min, followed by 7 cycles of 94°C for 30 sec, 65° to 59°C for 30 sec (decreased by 1°C intervals per cycle), and 72°C for 30 sec, followed by 38 cycles of 90°C for 30 sec, 58°C for 30 sec, and 72°C for 30 sec, with a final 10 min at 72°C. The reactions were performed on an Applied Biosystems GeneAmp PCR System 9700 (Foster City, CA, USA) using 384-well plates (MJ Research, Waltham, MA). SLC6A4 SNPs were cycled on a DNA Engine Tetrad PTC-225 thermal cycler in 384-well plates (MJ Research, Waltham, MA). PCR conditions for SLC6A4 SNPs 9 and 11 were 1.5 mM magnesium with the following protocol: 94°C for 3 min, followed by 45 cycles of 90°C for 30 sec, 55°C for 30 sec, and 72°C for 30 sec, with a final 10 min at 72°C. The excess primers and deoxynucleotides in the PCR reaction were then degraded by adding a 0.2µl of 10X PCR Clean-Up Reagent (containing a mixture of shrimp alkaline phosphatase and exonuclease I) and 1.8µl of PCR Clean-Up Dilution Buffer to each 5µl PCR reaction (PerkinElmer, Boston, MA, USA). The mixture was then incubated at 37°C for 60 min, followed by inactivation for 15 min at 80°C. The final step was the addition of a 13µl solution containing a final concentration of 0.38µM TDI probe (Table 2.1), 2µl of 10X TDI Reaction Buffer, 0.5µl of AcycloTerminator Mix (containing R110 and TAMRA labeled AcycloTerminators, corresponding to the polymorphic base), and 0.025µl of AcycloPol DNA polymerase (PerkinElmer). This mixture was cycled at 95°C for 2 min, followed by 25 cycles of 94°C for 15 sec and 55°C for 30 sec. Following template-directed incorporation, fluorescence polarization

SNP ID	dbSNP rs#	Position	Alleles	Allele freq.	Size	Forward / Reverse / FP Probe
HTR1A-1	rs968555	5'	G/T	3/97	248	catgtgttgtttgacacaattctta
						gatttgtgaaggtatctatttccactt
						aaagctgaattatctaaaattaaacttttgaaa
HTR1A-2	rs6295	5'	C/G	52/48	94	gcgagaacggaggtagcttt
						ggtgaacagtcctgggtcag
						ggaagaagaccgagtgtgtcttc
HTR1A-3	rs6294	Exon (S)	A/G	2/98	173	gacctcatggtgtcggtgtt
						gtgatggcccagtacctgtc
						atggccgcgctgtatcaggt
HTR1A-4	rs1800044	Exon (S)	G/T	99/1	238	tcgctcacttggcttattgg
						cggtcttctccacctttttg
						gttctctatgggcgcatattcc
HTR1A-5	rs878567	3'	C/T	50/50	217	aagcgacattggctcagact
						ttcccaaacctcaagtccaa
						cctgtatcatcagttttgatcccag
HTR1A-6	rs749098	3'	C/G	73/27	236	attgcaaaaattgccagtga
						ttcactgcagacccttctca
						agagctgtcctttcactttcttaattataaa
HTR1A-7	rs749099	3'	A/G	50/50	250	caaaccccaaatttgctcat
						aaagcatcaggcactcttttg
						ccatttatttgtgtcttttacagaattgt
HTR1A-8	rs1423691	3'	A/G	50/50	152	taaccogaaagggtcttgg
						ccaccctgttgcaactcttt
						tcagaatgaggagagaatcattaacc
HTR1A-9	rs970453	3'	A/G	49/51	197	gcaggacttggtgtctggat
						ctgccatctggatttggaat
						cttttgcagcttcatcggtaaac
HTR1A-10	rs1364043	3'	G/T	27/73	167	tttgaagagggcacaattcc
						aagcgaactcaaacagcaaaa
						ccattcttaatacactacttaacatggtatttt
HTR2A-1	rs6311	5'	C/T	55/45	208	atggcctttgtgcagattc
						ctagccaccctgagcctatg
						cctcggagtgctgtgagtgtc
HTR2A-2	rs6312	5'	C/T	8/92	236	ggccaagcatgatttcaaac
						gctcttgcatgcagtttttg
						tgagaacttacatttgtcttcagggt
HTR2A-3	rs6313	Exon (S)	A/G	45/55	295	acccttcacaggaaaggttg
						cagcatgtacaccagcctca
						tgcatcagaagtgttagcttctcc
HTR2A-4	rs6304	Exon (NS)	C/T	2/98	218	ttcagaaagcacgaactgtca
						ggatttacctggacgtgctc
						cctactgatatggtccaaacagcaa
HTR2A-5	rs6305	Exon (S)	A/G	2/98	218	ttcagaaagcacgaactgtca
						ggatttacctggacgtgctc
						ttctggatggcgacgtagcg
HTR2A-6	rs2025296	Intron	C/T	91/9	233	tcataaaccaaccaactttgtca
						ttttgtttgctttgtgtgtgg
						agtctagctggaattttaaaatatgatctaac
HTR2A-7	rs927544	Intron	A/G	74/26	161	ctgggaatgtcctccagtgt
						agcatgctcatttaggtccaa
						tcaagcattttttttccagaagatac
HTR2A-8	rs1928039	Intron	C/T	4/96	153	cagcagatgggatctggttt
						aatgccccttaattcccatc
						cctgcatttcatgcagtttcct
HTR2A-9	rs666693	Intron	A/G	12/88	249	cgtgcaaaaaggacacatga
						atattctcagggcccattcc
						tgagaagcactgcctacactatca
HTR2A-10	rs2770296	Intron	C/T	26/74	230	aggcttaccgagaaagctga
						tcaaagccaggtcttgtgact
						ctgtgcaatcaactcaggcct
HTR2A-11	rs659734	Intron	A/G	93/7	222	gcaggaatggaaagctgact
						cacgtcagcccaagtttaca
						ataatagctggtaggaaattgaactgaa
HTR2A-12	rs2246127	Intron	C/T	40/60	233	aagcaaaacaatccctcgtaga
						cttcaaaaccctgctgcatt
						cccacttgctttgttcagaaaaa

Table 2.1. Pharmacodynamic candidate gene SNP assay descriptions.

46

SNP ID	dbSNP rs#	Position	Alleles	Allele freq.	Size	Forward / Reverse / FP Probe
HTR2A-13	rs619549	Intron	A/G	1/99	189	gtcccagtcatcggtagcat tctcctgaaagcccatcact ttttgctttggaatattatcaaatagc
HTR2A-14	rs1923884	Intron	A/G	14/86	202	tctcatcttggccttgctct gcccaggggcactaatctat tggtacaaatagtgtcagctgatcag
HTR2A-15	rs1923882	Intron	C/T	70/30	195	cagcctgggagaaaaagtca gatggcaagagtgaggcagt catattatcagcacactcagaattgtagaa
HTR2A-16	rs6314	Exon (NS)	A/G	10/90	250	ccacggcaactagcctatca ttcagtgtcagtacaaggaaaacaa gctattgtctttagaagcctcttcagaat
HTR2A-17	rs3125	3' UTR	C/G	18/82	165	ccaagcacacattttgtagca caactgtggaaggcacactg agtctagtggaaccaacgatcatatct
HTR2C-1	rs540285	5'	C/T	59/41	202	gtgttccatcattgcctcag aagggtatcccaggcaaaa aatgagagtctcagcacacagca
HTR2C-2	rs527236	5'	A/G	23/77	249	aggcagatttgctgctgatt tcacttcaaaactgccagga aaaatttcagtaatgcaaatatttaaaaagtaat
HTR2C-3	rs493533	5'	C/T	61/39	174	gagatggcttcaggactgc tcattgctctattagccaacca tctatcatatttacccttttggaattgtg
HTR2C-4	Yuan C-759T	5'	C/T	85/15	172	gtgcatctgaggaaggaagc gcactaagagaccggtccaa ttggctcctcccctcatcc
HTR2C-5	rs518147	5' UTR	C/G	39/61	172	gtgcatctgaggaaggaagc gcactaagagaccggtccaa taggcgctctggtgcttgc
HTR2C-6	rs543229	Intron	C/T	25/75	152	aagcacccccaaatcctacct cctggggagggaagaaaata tgcaatcaacaagccttatcca
HTR2C-7	rs538680	Intron	C/T	98/2	222	ttagctgagagggatgacg tttcccctcaatttttcaagg aggcttgactcaattataatgttgga
HTR2C-8	rs556677	Intron	C/T	76/24	226	atatggtggctgttgcactg aaggccttctggtccctaaa agctattagaaagcctttagaactgcat
HTR2C-9	rs498177	Intron	A/G	55/45	249	ccacagtactggacttctccaa tgatctgagcccaggtagaaa gttatttcagggtagaaagaccatacttg
HTR2C-10	rs1023574	Intron	C/G	62/38	201	gccaatacggcttacatttca aaataagaaagcttagccaggaaa ggtattcatttagtaacaccatatttcaattat
HTR2C-11	rs2192371	Intron	A/G	61/39	160	tgggatcagaccaagttacca ctccaatatgggctgaaaaca gtctggtaaaccacctgtctaatctatta
HTR2C-12	rs2192372	Intron	A/G	39/61	172	tccataacccgattgctctt tctgaaggcaattcaagcaa ccagcaaatatttagacatgtgacatttt
HTR2C-13	rs2248440	Intron	C/T	77/23	249	gcaagccatttatgcagattt tctctccccagaaaaggatga gcaagctaccaagcaaagttatctttt
HTR2C-14	rs2428727	Intron	C/T	23/77	229	ccctttacggcagtcctaca ggcccatcttgagtgtcatt ggctatatactaagttggcacaggc
HTR2C-15	rs6318	Exon (NS)	C/G	77/23	186	aatttgaagcgtccaccatc gttgtttgcatgagcaacg gctactgggctcacagaaatatca
HTR2C-16	rs2497527	Intron	G/T	19/81	243	tttctggaggacccttcctt tggaaattggcagtcattca tgtagtttaatcctgcaaagctacatagat
HTR2C-17	rs2497522	Intron	C/T	77/23	154	tttttgggtgaatgcctgag cccttcacaaagtccctctg tcaagatcagccctgtggaata

Table 2.1 (con't). Pharmacodynamic candidate gene SNP assay descriptions.

47

SNP ID	dbSNP rs#	Position	Alleles	Allele freq.	Size	Forward / Reverse / FP Probe
HTR2C-18	rs2428698	Intron	C/T	81/19	172	cacctcggaaaataccattga cataacagaaaatgtttggcaga tgacagatgaactgacatggcac
HTR2C-19	rs1414334	Intron	C/G	24/76	214	cagggataaaattggcctca tcacacacaggccatgagat gcttatctacagtgactttgctaccct
HTR2C-20	rs1360851	Intron	A/C	79/21	199	tgctcaaaattccacacagaa gatggctgggctgagtctaa gtaaaatgtagagttgggagatatgcagt
HTR2C-21	rs1360852	Intron	C/T	78/22	199	tgctcaaaattccacacagaa gatggctgggctgagtctaa gaaaagattctctttttagcaagggtttt
HTR2C-22	rs1414324	3'	C/T	77/23	154	tattatttgccagccgcttc gatgctggattgagaacacattt ccattcacctctgtgtgatttga
HTR2C-23	rs1414327	3'	A/G	22/78	250	caatacagcagttccttgcaca tgctgccctatgaaaaaggt tcaacatggtttctttataacatcgatac
HTR2C-24	rs2310797	3'	C/T	23/77	219	tggggctttaatccctatctg caccctcgataactggcatt aactcacttgcctagggtcacag
HTR2C-25	rs1335617	3'	C/T	25/75	189	tggagctttgtctcctcagc cagggacaaacagatcagca ttttaagttttgtcatcccaacctta
MAOA-1	rs2310820	5'	G/T	73/27	190	cttggctggcagagacttttc ggagaaacggttcagaggaa aaactttatctctctttctgaaaggaaac
MAOA-2	rs1181275	5'	A/G	9/91	267	atccctaatgggagttgcac aagagtgaaacgccatctcaa ttttcaaaaatatataggaaggataaatc
MAOA-3	rs1465107	Intron	C/T	71/29	298	tttgccattcaaatcagcag tgaagggttaaggtttaagttatttagg ggagctcagaaatcttttgtaatgtaataac
MAOA-4	rs1465108	Intron	A/G	31/69	298	tttgccattcaaatcagcag tgaagggttaaggtttaagttatttagg gtaaacatgcaaactgaaacattagc
MAOA-5	rs2179098	Intron	C/T	99/1	230	ctcccaaactgctgggatta tggcatctgtgaaagaggaa ttaagatagaaacaataatgagttcttctgg
MAOA-6	rs6323	Exon	A/C	69/31	250	tgaggaaattgacagaccaaga ccagagcttccagcagagag aatgacagctcccattggaag
MAOA-7	rs979606	Intron	C/T	30/70	373	aagaaatggggattttgacaac caaaaggccattgcttggta cttttgttaaagcaacgatattattgact
MAOA-8	rs979605	Intron	A/G	31/69	373	aagaaatggggattttgacaac caaaaggccattgcttggta caaatttaaaaggaaaagcagagttca
TPH1-1	Rotondo T-7180G	5'	A/C	66/34	248	attcactaatgttgcaggatacaaa aggattcttccgatccatga caaaggagtgaaagatctctacaatga
TPH1-2	Rotondo T-7065C	5'	C/T	65/35	248	attcactaatgttgcaggatacaaa aggattcttccgatccatga tgttcaccattggcatacagaaa
TPH1-3	Rotondo T-5806G	5'	G/T	66/34	248	gccgtccttaaccacacaag gttgctctgcctcaaggaat tattaaatagcccagaagcacagaga
TPH1-4	rs652458	5'	C/T	43/57	217	tgccctaggaattaggcattt ggggtctttgtctatttgtttgc ttatatcataaagcaactttccacatg
TPH1-5	rs623580	5'	A/T	30/70	226	tcagggatggcctcagataa cttgcctagatggatttgcag agtatgggcgacgttgtccta
TPH1-6	rs685249	Intron	A/C	55/45	187	gggagggaggtggtatcagt acataccatattctcagtcccactc caacctcttttaactatttctggtcgtt

Table 2.1 (con't). Pharmacodynamic candidate gene SNP assay descriptions.

SNP ID	dbSNP rs#	Position	Alleles	Allele freq.	Size	Forward / Reverse / FP Probe
TPH1-7	rs684302	Intron	A/G	45/55	220	ggaatgaagagagatggagca cccagtccttccaaatctga aataaaatacctgtatgtcttcttccatca
TPH1-8	rs211107	Intron	G/T	55/45	229	gatgggggtgctctgtgtat ttcttcgcagcccttaccta ggagattatctgctctaaccttctcatt
TPH1-9	rs172423	Intron	C/T	21/79	208	gggacttggggaagtagctc ttcactcgaggcaaaagaca aatagcagtcctgattacacctcaaata
TPH1-10	rs211105	Intron	A/C	79/21	214	tcaggttgatgtctaagtttttgga agatcaaggtggcaaagacaa atttctaagatcttttccatcggc
TPH1-11	rs2056246	Intron	A/C	45/55	262	gctctttttccaagggtgagg accatgctcagccattttgt acaagatatagtcaaatgattaaggaaaaaa
TPH1-12	rs1607395	Intron	A/G	55/45	210	tgctttgttttctccacatatggta gaggcataaacaaagggtaagg tttgttcctttagttctttatatttgtttg
TPH1-13	rs2237907	Intron	C/G	55/45	170	tgcagatatccccttccaac gatttggaggaaacgctttg gctgatctcttagggtctggagc
TPH1-14	rs1800532	Intron	G/T	55/45	221	tttcccccactggaatacaa tttttggtgtgcgaggatta tccctatgctcagaatagcagcta
TPH1-15	rs1799913	Intron	G/T	55/45	164	accgttgccagtttttgaac cactgcagcgtgacaaactt agttcatggcaggtatctctgaaa
TPH1-16	rs211102	Intron	A/G	17/83	151	actctgctccagcttcttgc tcctgggagaaggacatctg agcacatcactcattttccatca
TPH1-17	rs1134530	3'	A/T	2/98	409	tttgcttacagtagatttccttgc catcagcttcctttcccagt ctaatcaactcttaagtatacatttgatggtaaa
TPH1-18	rs2108977	3'	C/T	60/40	409	tttgcttacagtagatttccttgc catcagcttcctttcccagt ctataaatcagataatcaatatttcaaatgattc
TPH1-19	rs521318	3'	C/T	3/97	291	agttgtggattataaggctgtgc ttggttgcaaggaaatctactg cgttatcaaagttgtatgaaaataacca
TPH2-1	rs2129575	Intron	G/T	76/24	210	actggaaagcatttggcaag cagcaaggtcagtggttcct ggatcaatgcctggacactaaa
TPH2-2	rs1386488	Intron	G/T	21/79	229	tcctgtgaggcgaatttttc gtcgtggagaaaggacgaag cttctcatctgtcttaagcaccatg
TPH2-3	rs1843809	Intron	G/T	21/79	238	ttggggggctgttacaatgat catgaggttcatgggctacc aggccctgagctctactttaattat
TPH2-4	rs2171363	Intron	C/T	53/47	205	caaccgccaggtagaaatgt gggtaagggaatgggtgaat ccccacctttggtgtttctg
TPH2-5	rs1386492	Intron	A/G	75/25	216	ttgctgggcattagacttca ctgcgagaagtggagtaggg cctgggaggatggtgtaccac
TPH2-6	rs1386491	Intron	C/G	22/78	216	ttgctgggcattagacttca ctgcgagaagtggagtaggg ctgctgcccagtaagggtcc
TPH2-7	rs1843812	Intron	C/T	81/19	240	gaatcctcacttggggtctg cccctcacaagcctatttcc gtgaaatgatgtcactgtatgattcat
TPH2-8	rs1487281	Intron	G/T	19/81	214	tcctcaggcagaaggaccta aggcacattatccctccaca tgatctttggagagaaaaaagcttta
TPH2-9	rs1386497	Intron	G/T	22/78	209	caagagccacataccatcca ttgtttctgcaagtgggtca ggctggttggaatctgtggg

Table 2.1 (con't). Pharmacodynamic candidate gene SNP assay descriptions.

49

SNP ID	dbSNP rs#	Position	Alleles	Allele freq.	Size	Forward / Reverse / FP Probe
TPH2-10	rs1487284	Intron	A/G	24/76	242	aaagggcgaaattcattgtg
						ctctcagcatgagaaagtactggt
						gcttttggtggtcatgaatcac
TPH2-11	rs1487278	Intron	C/T	20/80	215	ggcccctggagagtttctta
						tctccaaggagaagctcgac
						cctctaactttcaacaactcacgtt
TPH2-12	rs1487276	Intron	C/T	78/22	173	gcaaagggtcatttggaaaa
						tgcaggtattttgcctttca
						aatgagtgagactgctgaatataaaactag
TPH2-13	rs1386487	Intron	G/T	34/66	247	gacagcgtgtttggatttca
						cctcccaaattgaagggtatc
						ggtctgagctatcatttctgttttg
TPH2-14	rs1872824	3'	A/G	31/69	215	gaatgttggtggtgctgaca
						gcaggtgaaccttttctgga
						cctctcatctccccaaatgc
SLC6A4-1	rs25533	5'	C/T	7/93	166	ctgcgagcgtgtgtgtgt
						cgtcactttgaggcgaataaa
						ccgtacgcggcccctccc
SLC6A4-2	rs2020934	Intron	C/T	53/47	125	tctgtgtgaagccactgagg
						ttgctcaatttgcacaaacc
						ggtggcagtgaccgttccaa
SLC6A4-3	rs2066713	Intron	C/T	62/38	104	ctctctacccaggcccaga
						actgctcactgctgctgcta
						gatggaccgcatttcccttc
SLC6A4-4	rs2020936	Intron	A/G	81/19	179	gctaggggctgtgtgtgtgt
						aaggccaggcagtagcataa
						gaaggatatgaattctgacaagagcg
SLC6A4-5	rs2020937	Intron	A/T	62/38	179	gctaggggctgtgtgtgtgt
						aaggccaggcagtagcataa
						tgttgggccctccrccaccc
SLC6A4-6	rs2020938	Intron	A/G	78/22	179	gctaggggctgtgtgtgtgt
						aaggccaggcagtagcataa
						accrcacttgttgggccctcc
SLC6A4-7	rs2020939	Intron	C/T	60/40	179	gctaggggctgtgtgtgtgt
						aaggccaggcagtagcataa
						tggyggagggcccaacaagtg
SLC6A4-8	rs25528	Intron	G/T	21/79	143	ccagagctgagctgacttcc
						gggagaagagtgtgcaggtt
						ctgatgctggggtggttggt
SLC6A4-9	rs6354	5' UTR	G/T	19/81	148	caccccagcatcagtaacct
						cactgctgctcaccatttgt
						gctaagcccttgttattctgcaa
SLC6A4-10	rs6355	Exon (NS)	C/G	99/1	151	agcagttccaagtcctggtg
						gtccacagcatagccaatca
						ggatagagtgccgtgtgtcatct
SLC6A4-11	rs2020942	Intron	A/G	35/65	114	cctgaggtctgtgcaaatca
						agcaaactctttggaggaagg
						cacatggtttattctcgagcc
SLC6A4-12	rs140699	Intron	A/G	1/99	127	taacaggccaacccctca
						actcctggaacactggcaac
						ctgaagaattttacacgtaagtgcac
SLC6A4-13	rs140700	Intron	C/T	89/11	110	gaggtgggtgaatggatgtc
						atccgatccctgtgtgactc
						tgaagaccttgagaaaggaggg
SLC6A4-14	rs717742	Intron	A/T	79/21	137	ggttagcctggaactcctga
						catgcccttcggttttgt
						ctcttattattttatatacaggagcgc
SLC6A4-15	rs140701	Intron	A/G	42/58	139	agtgtgaggacgcacttggt
						agaggaggaggtggttgaca
						cacacataaggtcttgtgatgagaatt
SLC6A4-16	rs6353	Exon (S)	C/T	99/1	148	agaagcgatagccaacatgc
						gctgagtcctcctcctttcc
						atttcccctccatttcctcac
SLC6A4-17	rs1042173	3' UTR	A/C	56/44	130	aaactgcgtaggagagaacagg
						cttcctttcctgatgccaca
						aggttctagtagattccagcaataaaatt

Table 2.1 (con't). Pharmacodynamic candidate gene SNP assay descriptions.

The following SNPs were not polymorphic in our sample:	FP-TDI assays could not be developed for the following assays:
rs3033664	rs918643
rs1800043	rs1328685
rs1800042	rs1805055
rs1048281	rs6308
rs968554	rs1048952
rs1800045	rs505971
rs1800041	rs2376488
rs1799920	rs2497541
rs1799921	rs2310883
rs2149433	rs3027393
rs2070038	rs1801291
rs1058576	rs593414
rs1058573	Rotondo (1999) G-6526A
Yuan (2000) G-995A	rs2732333
rs2228669	rs2468922
rs3027394	rs2732330
rs2283726	rs2468912
rs1799835	rs2468913
rs1800465	rs25530
rs1803986	rs25531
rs3027408	rs25532
rs1133758	rs956304
rs211100	rs745706
rs211101	
rs490895	
rs503964	
rs2887148	
rs2887147	
rs1007023	
rs2468918	
rs6352	
rs140702	

Table 2.1 (con't). Pharmacodynamic gene SNP assay descriptions. Shown are all SNPs investigated in this current study. Position column indicates region of gene where SNP is located, according to UCSC genome browser (http://genome.ucsc.edu). Interrogated shows acycloterminators used for assay, and underlined is the ancestral allele, as inferred by genotyping primate DNA samples (not performed on *SLC6A4* variants). Allele frequency is given in same order as interrogated SNP alleles. Size of the PCR product is shown, as well as the forward, reverse and FP probe sequences in descending order. For SNPs without an assigned dbSNP ID, references are given for the following manuscripts: Yuan (34) and Rotondo (35).

was read using a Victor2 1420 Multilabel Counter (PerkinElmer). For the *SLC6A4*
SNPs, the genotypes were read using a TECAN Ultra plate reader (TECAN-US,
Research Triangle Park, NC). Data output is expressed in dimensionless units, mP, as
previously described (31;36).

2.2.3 SSRI pharmacodynamic gene repeat polymorphism genotyping. PCR
amplification of the VNTR in the upstream regulatory region of MAOA was carried
out using the primers listed in Table 2.2. Amplifications were performed in a final
volume of 10µl containing 20ng of genomic DNA template, 50µM dNTPs, 1M
anhydrous betaine, 50 mM KCl, 20mM Tris-HCl (pH 8.4), 1.5 mM $MgCl_2$, and 0.5
units Platinum Taq DNA polymerase. Samples were denatured at 95°C for 4 min,
followed by 35 cycles of 95°C for 1 min, 62°C for 1 min, and 72°C for 1 min, with a
final 10 min step at 72°C (37). PCR products were separated on an ABI Prism 3700
DNA Analyzer and alleles were scored using Genotyper 3.5 NT software (Applied
Biosystems).

PCR amplification of the tandem repeat polymorphisms in the upstream
regulatory region (5-HTTLPR) and intron 4 (Intron 2 VNTR) of SLC6A4 was carried
out with fluorescent dye-labeled primers listed in Table 2.2, as was amplification of a
simple sequence repeat in intron 9 (Intron 7 [GAAA]n). Of note, marker names are
keyed to traditional names for continuity with the literature, despite the misnaming
due to the discovery of additional non-coding exons. For these polymorphisms,
amplification was performed in a final volume of 5µl containing 20ng of genomic
DNA template, 50µM nucleotide mix (i.e., 50 µM each of dATP, dCTP, dTTP, and
25 µM each of dGTP and 7- deaza-dGTP), 1M anhydrous betaine, 5% DMSO, 50
mM KCl, 20 mM Tris-HCl (pH 8.4), 1.83 mM $MgCl_2$, 200 nM primers, and 0.25
units Platinum Taq DNA polymerase. Samples were denatured at 95°C for 5 min,

52

Gene	Polymorphism	Forward	Reverse	Size
SLC6A4	5-HTTLPR	atgccagcacctaacccctaatgt	ggaccgcaaggtgggcggga	418
SLC6A4	Intron 2 VNTR	tgttcctagtcttacgccagtg	cagaatggagggggtcagta	311
SLC6A4	Intron 7 (GAAA)n	accgcaccccgtctctctcttt	acacctgtaagcacagccacttg	269
MAOA	MAOA VNTR	acagcctgaccgtggagaag	gaacggacggctccattcgga	323

Table 2.2. Pharmacodynamic gene repeat polymorphism assay descriptions. Shown are the primers for all repeat (VNTR) polymorphisms investigated in this current study. Size represents size of amplicon in base pairs according to the sequence of the associated clone.

followed by 40 cycles of 95°C for 30 sec, 61°C for 30 sec, and 72°C for 1 min, with a

final 6 min step at 72°C. For the Intron 2 VNTR, amplification was performed in a

final volume of 5 μl containing 20 ng of genomic DNA template, 50 μM dNTPs, 1M

anhydrous betaine, 5% DMSO, 50 mM KCl, 20 mM Tris-HCl (pH 8.4), 1.5 mM

MgCl2, 300 nM primers, and 0.25 units Platinum Taq DNA polymerase. Samples

were denatured at 95°C for 5 min, followed by 35 cycles of 95°C for 30 sec, 56°C for

30 sec, and 72°C for 40 sec, with a final 6 min step at 72°C (38). Intron 7 (GAAA)n

was amplified using the same conditions and cycling protocol described above for

SNPs. PCR products for all three *SLC6A4* repeat polymorphisms were separated on

an ABI Prism 3100 DNA Analyzer and alleles were scored using Genotyper 3.5 NT

software (Applied Biosystems).

2.2.4 Genomic control SNP genotyping. In order to correct for any population

stratification within the sample collection, the method of genomic control (GC) was

used. A collection of 20 unlinked C/T SNPs were chosen randomly throughout the

genome (Table 2.3). They were chosen from a collection of 18,150 SNPs assayed

using a pooled sequencing strategy by Dr. Pui-Yan Kwok for the Allele Frequency

Project of the SNP Consortium (http://snp.cshl.org/allele_frequency_project/).

Candidate SNPs were then chosen by iterative elimination if the SNP a) failed in the 3

populations tested (Caucasian, African-American, Asian), b) was non-polymorphic in

Caucasians, the population, and f) was a non-C/T SNP. This yielded 1,423 SNPs

eligible for use. Of these, SNPs were chosen at random and were analyzed

bioinformatically to determine chromosomal location. This process was stopped

when at least two SNPs were localized to each of the 22 autosomes. Then the genome

was essentially divided into 20 segments, and SNPs were chosen to fit into each of

these segments. Naturally, very large chromosomes would be over-represented due to

Location	SNP ID	Freq (Cau)	Freq (AA)	Freq (Asian)	Size	Forward / Reverse / FP Probe
1p31	rs997532	0.70	0.80	0.35	144	tcattcgtcacatcctgatttt
						gcccaggcttctgttttaca
						tcaattaaaatcatagccattcttaatttca
1q42	rs734551	0.50	0.35	0.50	99	ccccagagaaacggaacat
						caatttggagtcgattcctgt
						aacttggactttgcaacatctttt
2p11	rs735738	0.65	0.30	0.10	107	aggttcattctggacaagcaa
						tatcgggggtcccttttaat
						caactctgcataagttcctgaaca
2p23	rs734693	0.30	0.40	0.35	110	cttaggccaatggggaaact
						gacactcagcatgccaggta
						gggaaggtgacccaagtgga
3p24	rs952134	0.30	0.50	0.40	96	ctcatctgcaggtcccactg
						ccttgcagggcattaggtat
						tgatctattaaagaacagaaccaatatagagata
4p12	rs728292	0.45	0.50	1.00	98	cactgtgcctttccagacct
						accccccacttcacattctt
						tcatatcctttcagaatgaaggga
5q13	rs28137	0.57	0.74	0.47	141	agcgtcagtttactccactcg
						accctactcccacagctaagaa
						tttcaaaatcactactctataatttcaagaaa
6q27	rs1123365	0.50	0.60	0.55	138	cacaggggtgtgaaattcct
						ttccaacatttggcaaacaa
						acccgttacgtccccaagc
7q31	rs1343903	0.70	0.70	0.60	300	caggcacataaagcccattt
						tcttcatctggccatggaat
						aatttttcatgttttataggaattatttctatct
8q23	rs722740	0.40	0.25	0.50	99	gcagcctgagatctagctttg
						gcagtcctgtcctcagcatt
						ttctggtttgtttatgataacttgcc
9p22	rs718623	0.37	0.51	0.11	121	tgatatgccaatcaaacacaatct
						aaggaagtaaggcaaccagga
						gctagtggtgttctggtattagtcaca
10q22	rs768498	0.50	0.68	0.90	131	tgagagggatttgggtgtgt
						tcccagactttctggctttc
						gcattttaacttcctcgttcctgt
11p11	rs730129	0.61	0.53	N	132	agccatgaagaaggtggaca
						ccctctggatcatgagctgt
						gggaaccgcaccctctcctc
12q13	rs998820	0.65	0.50	0.84	97	ggctcagcttgtctttccac
						caaagggacccaggaataca
						aaagggagagagcattgtttcc
13q14	rs730924	0.45	0.60	0.85	109	ctatctctgagaatgaatggagacc
						gttgaggcgacagaagtcct
						caagtacctacctgatacgaacaaaatt
14q32	rs1005788	0.33	0.57	0.55	105	gaaggtggaagaagctgtgg
						ccgtggacctcactggataa
						tcattgagatgctggctcaag
15q13	rs883473	0.50	0.25	0.25	117	gcccaaggtcactctgtgat
						tgactttgttctgccgaagtt
						ccaagtctaaaggaagcagcaga
16p12	rs24656	0.50	0.85	0.20	107	cctgagcatggatgggaata
						tggagcggataattaccaa
						gtgggaaacaagtcaatcaggaaca
17q24	rs719615	0.60	0.80	0.50	166	ctagcaaatggccaatcctg
						aaataatgttccacagaaaactaaagg
						aatgttcaagaaaatatattctatttccca
20q13	rs47223	0.60	0.62	0.68	101	gcacaaagccaacagtcctt
						cttgacaaggccgtcaattt
						gaaaagtgatggaaacgccc

Table 2.3. Genomic control SNP assay descriptions. Shown are the 20 SNPs used for the genomic control procedure. Listed are the chromosomal locations, as well as the dbSNP ID, and the allele frequency in Caucasian, African-American, and Asian samples. PCR amplicon size and primer and FP probe sequences are also shown. predominant group in this study, c) was non-polymorphic in the 3 populations, d) had minor allele frequency <0.3 in Caucasians, e) failed in African-American

the proportion of the genome found on those chromosomes. SNPs near genes are over-represented, with 11 occurring in non-gene regions and 9 occurring in the introns of known genes. There were no exonic SNPs in this group. SNPs were limited to C/T SNPs based on laboratory convenience and uniformity. These SNPs were genotyped using FP-TDI, as described above.

2.2.5 Statistical analysis. Single point association tests were performed via logistic regression using the statistical package R 1.6.1 (39). Alleles were coded as 0, 1, or 2 corresponding to the presence of 0, 1, or 2 copies of the rare allele. This coding scheme was chosen because of its robustness to departure from the true additive genetic model (40). For each SNP, three phenotypic comparisons were made based on the results from the response pattern analysis described in the Sample description. The comparisons made were: (1) all responders (specific and non-specific) versus non-responders, (2) specific responders versus both non-specific responders and non-responders, and (3) specific responders versus non-specific responders. Empirical p-values were obtained based on 100,000 simulations using the CLUMP computer program (41). This program holds the marginal allele frequencies constant and permutes the cell counts in a contingency table. For each SNP with nominally significant association, odds ratio estimates and 95% confidence intervals (CI) were computed, comparing carriers of the rare allele to non-carriers. Haplotypes using all markers from each gene were constructed and frequencies estimated using an Expectation Maximization (EM) algorithm in the Arlequin 2.0 program (42). For selection of "tag" SNPs (htSNPs), haplotype frequency estimations for each gene region were entered into the SNPtagger program (43). A "coverage value" of 80% was set in order to capture the major haplotype diversity while excluding the extremely rare haplotypes. Haplotype frequency differences were then tested for significance using the three response phenotype comparisons listed above with the CLUMP computer program (41)

Hardy-Weinberg Equilibrium (HWE) was determined for each SNP using the Arlequin 2.0 program (42). Linkage disequilibrium across each candidate gene was assessed using the computer program GOLD (44). For MAOA and HTR2C, the X-linked option was chosen. We accounted for population stratification through the use of GC (45). This was determined by adjusting the single point χ^2 statistic by a correction factor λ. Briefly, the χ^2 statistic is generated for each GC SNP. These numbers are then averaged, generating λ. The χ^2 for each candidate association test is computed and then divided by λ, approximating a χ^2 with one degree of freedom. The significance level was set at $p < 0.05$ after GC correction. This significance threshold, while liberal given the number of SNPs that we tested, reflects our acknowledgment of the limited statistical power of this sample as well as the fact that this study is intended to be hypothesis generating as opposed to a strict replication or validation of previously suspected variants.

2.3 Results

2.3.1 Single locus association results. In our primary phenotypic comparison, response versus non-response to fluoxetine, three SNPs in the TPH1 gene were significantly associated (p<0.05) (Table 2.4). Odds ratio estimates indicated a protective effect, i.e., carriers of the rare allele were less likely to respond to treatment. However, both of the previously studied A218C and A779C *TPH1* SNPs (22) did not reach significance in our study. A single *SLC6A4* SNP showed nominally significant association to treatment response (p=0.037). None of the SNPs investigated in the *TPH2, HTR1A, HTR2A, HTR2C*, or *MAOA* gene region reached significance in this phenotypic comparison.

In an effort to utilize detailed clinical information in order to provide more precise phenotypic definitions, we attempted to further delineate treatment response phenotypes using clinical data. We performed two such alternative phenotypic comparisons involving subgroups of the patients by specificity of response type as classified through use of pattern analysis. The first comparison is based on the hypothesis that specific responders differ genetically from all other subjects. The second comparison is a variation of this hypothesis: among responders, specific responders differ genetically from non-responders. In the specific response vs. all others (non-specific response and non-response) comparison, one SNP in the *HTR2A* gene and three SNPs in the *TPH2* gene led to significant associations (Table 2.4). None of the SNPs tested in the *HTR1A, HTR2C, SLC6A4, TPH1*, or *MAOA* gene regions yielded significant association with this phenotypic comparison.

In our third phenotypic comparison, specific response vs. non-specific response, both the *HTR2A* and the *MAOA* gene regions contained significantly associated SNPs. In the *HTR2A* gene region, 3 SNPs located at the 3' end of the coding region showed significant negative associations (Table 2.4). While the *MAOA*-VNTR failed to show significance in this study, two SNPs in the *MAOA* gene did show nominal significance. None of the SNPs studied in the *HTR1A, HTR2C, SLC6A4, TPH1*, or *TPH2* gene regions had significant association using this phenotypic comparison.

2.3.2 Pharmacodynamic gene haplotype association results. To examine interaction of alleles from different SNPs within a gene, haplotypes (i.e., those including information from all markers at the locus) were inferred and tested for

Gene	SNP	R vs NR		S vs NS and NR		S vs NS		Minor allele frequencies (%)		
		p-value	Odds Ratio* (95% CI)	p-value	Odds Ratio* (95% CI)	p-value	Odds Ratio* (95% CI)	R vs NR	S vs NS and NR	S vs NS
SLC6A4	1	0.037	0.33 (0.08 - 1.35)	-	-	-	-	5/16	-	-
TPH1	1	0.022	0.41 (0.11 - 1.37)	-	-	-	-	30/50	-	-
TPH1	2	0.035	0.43 (0.12 - 1.45)	-	-	-	-	31/50	-	-
TPH1	3	0.022	0.41 (0.11 - 1.37)	-	-	-	-	30/50	-	-
HTR2A	15	-	-	0.016	0.34 (0.13 - 0.86)	0.0008	0.17 (0.04 - 0.66)	-	23/40	23/53
HTR2A	16	-	-	-	-	0.020	0.30 (0.08 - 1.15)	-	-	8/23
HTR2A	17	-	-	-	-	0.026	0.27 (0.08 - 0.87)	-	-	13/30
TPH2	3	-	-	0.020	2.60 (0.96 - 7.17)	-	-	-	27/13	-
TPH2	5	-	-	0.042	2.33 (0.92 - 6.02)	-	-	-	31/17	-
TPH2	12	-	-	0.035	3.00 (1.11 - 8.25)	-	-	-	27/14	-
MAOA	4	-	-	-	-	0.027	0.34 (0.10 - 1.09)	-	-	27/50
MAOA	6	-	-	-	-	0.049	0.27 (0.08 - 0.90)	-	-	27/46

Table 2.4. Single locus association results. SNPs with an unadjusted permutation p-value <0.05 are shown. Minor allele frequencies for each phenotype classification (e.g., R % / NR %) are displayed. R = response; NR = non-response; S = specific response; NS = nonspecific response.

*Odds ratios compare carrier of rare allele relative to non-carrier. 95% confidence intervals (CIs) are also shown for the odds ratios.

association using the three phenotypic comparisons (Table 2.5). Initially, all SNPs were considered and included in haplotype construction for each gene. Haplotypes for three genes (*TPH2*, *SLC6A4*, and *HTR2A*) were significantly associated with the specific response versus all others phenotype, and haplotypes for *MAOA*, *SLC6A4*, and *HTR2A* were associated with the specific responder versus non-specific responder comparison. For example, full length haplotypes constructed with all 17 *HTR2A* SNPs examined in this study and tested using the specific response versus all other subjects comparison showed significant association (p=0.011). When the phenotypic comparison was narrowed to specific responder versus non-specific responder, *HTR2A* haplotypes were still associated with specific response (p=0.001). In general, positive haplotype association results followed the positive single locus results, however, full length haplotype testing of *TPH1* failed to reach significance in the response vs. non-response comparison.

Knowledge of extensive LD and the existence of haplotype blocks in the human genome suggest that a limited number of SNPs may capture a substantial amount of haplotypic diversity in a population (46). We sought to determine if a subset of the SNPs we have genotyped in our sample could be used to test for association between multi-marker haplotypes and our clinical phenotypes. One approach to accomplish this is to use haplotype tag SNPs (htSNPs), as identified using the SNPtagger program (43). We chose a coverage value of 80%, as we wanted to capture the most common haplotypes and a number of the less common haplotypes, but exclude the substantial number of haplotypes estimated to occur one or fewer times in our sample.

After htSNPs yielding at least 80% coverage of the haplotypic diversity were identified in each gene region, haplotypes were constructed from genotypes of this

60

Gene	Phenotypic comparison	Total number of SNPs	p-value (all SNPs)	htSNPs required	htSNP number of haplotypes tagged	p-value (htSNP)
TPH2	R vs. NR	14	0.42	4	9	0.0005
TPH1	R vs. NR	19	0.39	2	4	0.0006
HTR2A	R vs. NR	17	0.67	9	22	0.004
TPH2	S vs. NS and NR	14	0.04	4	9	0.007
HTR2A	S vs. NS and NR	17	0.01	9	22	0.0001
SLC6A4	S vs. NS and NR	21	0.02	6	12	0.17
MAOA	S vs. NS	9	0.04	2	3	0.19
HTR2A	S vs. NS	17	0.001	9	22	0.0001
SLC6A4	S vs. NS	21	0.004	6	12	0.08

Table 2.5. Full length and htSNP haplotype analysis results. Total number of SNPs investigated in each gene are shown, along with the number of htSNPs needed to capture 80% of haplotype diversity in our sample population. Number of inferred haplotypes captured by the htSNP set are also shown. Only genes with significantly different (p<0.05) haplotype distributions between fluoxetine response phenotypes are shown, as determined using the CLUMP program.

smaller set of SNPs using Arlequin and tested for association to the phenotype using the CLUMP program. In general, the use of htSNPs to construct haplotypes led to more significant associations than using all of the SNPs screened, with the exception of the *SLC6A4* and *MAOA* genes (Table 2.5). We found that this procedure indicated that the majority of haplotypes could be captured with a limited number of SNPs. For example, we initially genotyped 19 SNPs in the *TPH1* gene region, but after haplotype frequency estimations were calculated it was apparent that only two SNPs were needed to capture the four most common haplotypes, which accounted for 87% (167/192) of the haplotypes seen in our study population. The use of htSNPs also implicated the *TPH1*, *TPH2* and *HTR2A* gene regions in the primary comparison, response vs. non-response, which were not significant when all possible SNPs were used for haplotype construction. For instance, the *TPH1* gene region, which contained six associated SNPs in the categorical response versus non-response comparison, was not significantly associated when all 19 SNPs were used to construct haplotypes (p=0.387). However, when only the two htSNPs were used to construct haplotypes, a positive association was seen (p=0.0006).

2.3.3 Assessment of population stratification using genomic control. There has been much debate about the role of population stratification in case-control studies with the attendant possibility of false positive associations, and less discussed, false negative findings (47). A number of approaches have been proposed to estimate the role of stratification using the genome itself to determine population heterogeneity (48;49). Here we use the genomic control (GC) approach of Devlin, in which anonymous markers from across the genome are genotyped in cases and controls, and the association test statistic is rescaled based upon the degree of observed stratification (45;48). We chose 20 SNPs distributed across the genome, and genotyped our sample for those SNPs, as described in the Methods. Allele frequency results for those SNPs are available on request. When comparing the response group vs. non-response group, GC analysis produced λ of 1.21, indicating perhaps a need to adjust the p-values for slight population stratification. However, since the stratification for this phenotype comparison was slight at best and we have limited statistical power, we did not adjust the test statistics. For the other two phenotypic comparisons made, specific response vs. all others and specific response vs. non-specific response, GC analysis yielded a λ of <1.0, indicating that the patient populations were not significantly stratified given the limits of the small sample size.

2.3.4 Assessment of linkage disequilibrium (LD). Levels of linkage disequilibrium were calculated for each gene region using genotypic data (Figure 2.3). As can be seen from the pairwise |D'| values shown in the figure, levels of LD were generally substantial, but variable between the gene regions screened. Although there is a trend for increased LD across smaller gene regions, this was not an absolute rule as one of the smaller gene regions (*HTR2A* – 63Kb) showed significantly less LD than the largest gene region (*HTR2C* – 395Kb).

2.3.5 Primate genotyping results. SNPs examined in all genes this study except for *SLC6A4* were also genotyped in 5 primate genomic DNA samples, four unrelated chimpanzees and one bonobo, using the same primers and conditions as used for the human genotyping. Of the 93 SNPs investigated in total, six failed to produce readable genotype results. Four SNPs had at least one heterozygotic chimpanzee sample, indicating present day variation within this species. There were 83 SNPs where the primate samples were all homozygous for the same allele, implicating it as the ancestral allele for humans (Table 2.1). The most frequent (major) SNP allele in

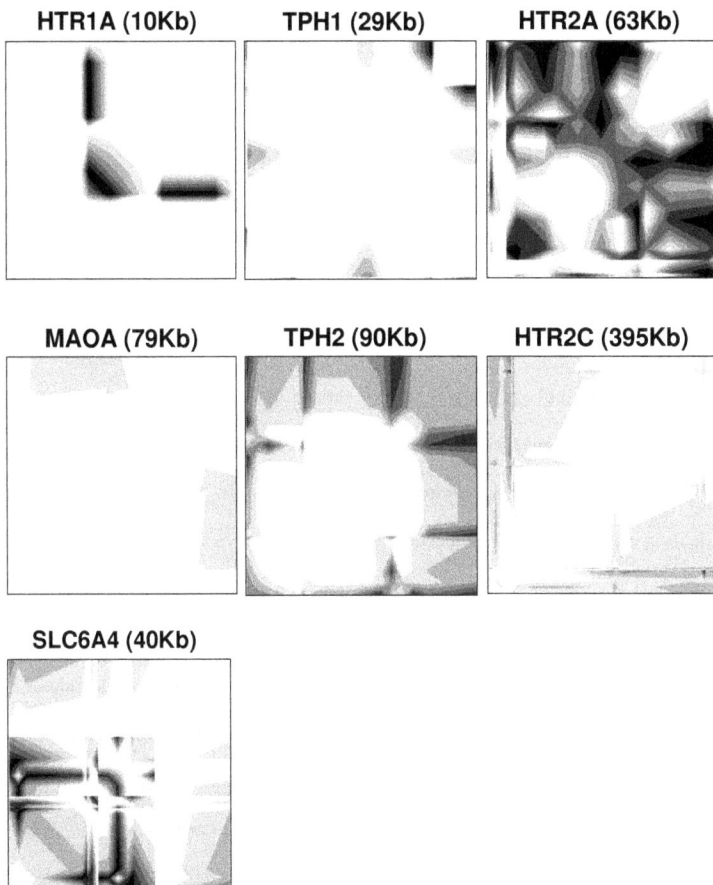

HTR1A (10Kb) **TPH1 (29Kb)** **HTR2A (63Kb)**

MAOA (79Kb) **TPH2 (90Kb)** **HTR2C (395Kb)**

SLC6A4 (40Kb)

Figure 2.3. Linkage disequilibrium plots. The above plots are the graphical outputs of linkage disequilibrium from the GOLD program. They represent the pairwise marker D' scores starting with the first marker in the lower left corner of each plot and continuing in the X and Y directions to the last marker. Lighter areas have high levels on LD, whereas darker areas indicate lower levels of LD.

our human population matched this presumed ancestral allele in 46 out of 83 cases (Figure 2.4).

2.4 Discussion

There has been much recent interest in the use of genetic variants for the prediction of medication treatment response (50). This interest is quite strong for the psychopharmacologic treatment of psychiatric disorders, which in general are still treated empirically, with an unacceptable rate of failure for first-line treatments. The recent collection of large amounts of DNA variants in the form of SNPs and inexpensive genotyping technologies make more comprehensive analyses of genetic variation in genes of interest for treatment response feasible. We have utilized these tools in order to perform an in-depth analysis of common variants in seven genes involved in serotonin function. We have genotyped a well-characterized sample of patients with unipolar Major Depressive Disorder at a number of SNPs within each gene, and tested for association to a treatment response phenotype using individual loci and multi-locus haplotypes. Using convergent analytic strategies, we found association between several of these genes and antidepressant response phenotype. For our primary phenotype, categorical response versus non-response, several *TPH1* SNPs were negatively associated with the phenotype. Odds ratios estimates indicated that carriers of the rare allele had a higher risk of not responding to treatment. This comparison also yielded a negative association to a single *SLC6A4* SNP. The location of this SNP, some 200 bases 5' to exon 1a, raises suspicion about a potential role in regulatory elements. But without biological evidence, it is premature to speculate on the function of this SNP. Our results differ in regard to a number of other studies in

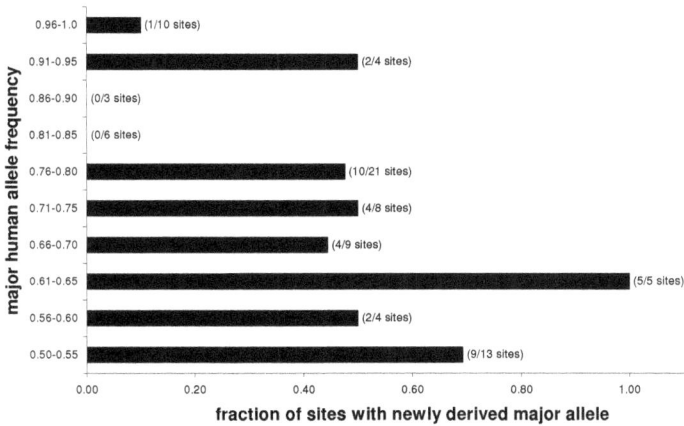

Figure 2.4. Putative ancestral allele state of SNPs interrogated. Correlations between human allele frequencies and putative ancestral allele state for the 83 SNPs which were monomorphic in our non-human primate samples. SNPs were binned into one of ten major allele frequency groupings as shown on the y-axis. The fraction of occurrences where the major human SNP allele corresponds to a newly derived human allele is shown on the x-axis.

which associations were found between response and 5-HTTLPR. It might be argued that perhaps our population differs from other Caucasian samples in which this association has been noted. However, for the *SLC6A4* promoter polymorphism, we observed population allele frequencies (short =0.43, long = 0.57) that were close to those found in other European American populations (51;52). Our own observations also closely match those reported in a recent study of 847 Caucasians in New Zealand, which revealed an allele frequency for the long allele of 0.57 (53). Likewise, the intron 2 VNTR allele frequencies (9 = 0.005, 10 = 0.390, 12 = 0.605) that we observed matched those seen in European Americans (54), although we did observe an under-representation of the rarer 9 allele when compared to Gelernter, *et al* (52). We observed association between our second phenotype, specific responders versus all other subjects, at two genes, *HTR2A* and *TPH2*. With this comparison, our data supported an increased risk of specific response of carriers of the less frequent *TPH2* allele, but decreased risk of carriers of the minor *HTR2A* allele. Finally, we observed negative associations between SNPs coming from *HTR2A* and *MAOA* and our third phenotype, specific responders versus non-specific responders. We are intrigued by the finding that in almost all cases in which we had significant association between a response phenotype and a SNP, it was carrier status of the minor allele that appeared to be associated with *non-response* or the *non-specific pattern of response*. Does this suggest that the default genetic and biological substrate for fluoxetine treatment leads to specific response, while the presence of less common alleles somehow degrades response or changes the specificity of the response? Given the limitations of this study, this speculation is premature, but nevertheless a potentially exciting observation.

We have attempted to analyze multiple genetic components of the serotonin pathway for their role in antidepressant response. The use of both single locus and haplotypic association is not novel, but it is still uncommon to see a coordinated investigation of multiple genes. It will be important to extend our findings by employing a joint analysis of the pathway, but such methods are currently in development or are untested.

Thus far, the vast majority of studies on serotonin pathway gene variants in antidepressant response have focused on single SNP associations. The use of haplotypes, or particular combinations of alleles observed in a population, has been shown both theoretically and empirically to be a powerful approach for the dissection of complex genetic traits (55-58). We found haplotypes associated with our response phenotypes for several of the genes we investigated. Further, using a haplotype SNP tagging approach, we were able to reduce the number of SNPs required to represent the majority of haplotypes, and generally noted even greater association between these htSNP haplotypes and phenotype. It has become commonplace to note that limited haplotypic diversity exists in many regions of the genome, and the seven genes we investigate proved to be no exception. The use of multiple SNPs also allows for estimation of linkage disequilibrium (LD) within a given gene, which provides useful information for association mapping, particularly for the selection of markers. We were not surprised to find extensive LD across the genes under examination here.

Accurate assessment of clinical response is essential in pharmacogenetic studies, as there is a need to limit the amount of phenotypic heterogeneity. This is particularly true with antidepressant therapy, as placebo response rates can be as high as 60% for patients with Major Depressive Disorder (29;59). Previous studies with serotonin pathway gene variants and SSRI antidepressant response have failed to address these concerns. It is reasonable to hypothesize that genetic factors may influence placebo response to antidepressants, given recent evidence showing that subjects homozygous for the long allele of the 5-HTTLPR were more likely to respond to placebo in a fluoxetine trial in 51 depressed subjects (60). In this study, we utilized a validated response pattern algorithm to classify patients as non-responders, specific responders, or placebo (non-specific) responders to fluoxetine (24;25;27). We were thus able to obtain a more precise assessment of clinical response phenotype, and potentially identify phenocopies. The use of pattern analysis to define response type reduced the amount of phenotypic heterogeneity in our comparison groups and was integral in uncovering some of our findings. Indeed, had we only investigated the most obvious phenotypic comparison, responders versus non-responders, we would have found negligible association between response and genotype. What is interesting in the current work is that we detected a number of differences between treatment populations using more precise phenotypic stratification, namely by trying to separate specific responders from non-specific responders. A number of our findings suggest that specific responders differ genetically from all others (i.e., from non-responders and non-specific responders) (*HTR2A*, *SLC6A4*, and *TPH2*). Similar findings indicate that even among responders, specific responders may differ at several candidate loci from non-specific responders (*HTR2A* and *MAOA*). This suggests that there may be heritable differences underlying the *nature* of response to fluoxetine. This is interesting in the context of imaging data that shows differential brain glucose metabolism in persons with depression administered placebo or fluoxetine (61). Specifically, hospitalized males receiving placebo or fluoxetine for unipolar depression underwent positron emission

69

tomography before and after six weeks of treatment. The authors found that placebo response was associated with specific regional changes in brain function. Remarkably, these regions showed overlap with changes seen in fluoxetine responders, but were not identical. Similar differences were seen using quantitative electroencephalography, suggesting different biological responses underlying specific response, non-specific response, or non-response to antidepressant medication (62). Although our methodology for assessing the placebo phenotype differs from that of Rausch *et al.* (60), it is interesting to note that our most positive findings for the serotonin transporter are seen when we attempted to dissect out placebo-responsive subjects in the work described here. Given the high placebo response rate for many antidepressants, it may prove necessary to control for non-specific responses in pharmacogenetic studies on antidepressant response.

An important issue that has been overlooked in many case-control association studies of antidepressant response (or association studies in general) is population stratification, or differences in allele frequencies between populations that may lead to spurious associations. One method that has been used to deal with population stratification is the use of ethnically matched cases and controls. However, a significant amount of "cryptic stratification" may still exist even after cases and control are carefully matched (63). We employed the method of genomic control (GC) to correct for any underlying stratification within our population. This method uses allele frequency data for a number of unlinked loci to quantitatively assess the degree of stratification present within the study population (45;64). This produces a correction factor which is used to adjust the critical level of significance required for a positive association at the candidate SNPs, thereby reducing the rate of false positives (45). In general, we found little evidence for population stratification in our sample, suggesting that the genetic differences detected between our phenotypic groups are unlikely to be due to ethnic stratification. Although our genomic control markers suggest minimal stratification, it is also possible that the sample size or number of markers may not be large enough to allow a more accurate estimation of stratification.

Genotyping of five primate samples gave insight into the evolutionary history of these polymorphic sites. Ancestral allele was inferred if the human SNP site was monomorphic across all non-human primate samples screened. A high fraction (37/83) of SNPs had discrepancy between the most common allele seen in humans and the most common allele from non-human primates. The correlation between human common allele state and ancestral allele state was similar to previous findings, indicating caution is in order when assigning ancestral allele state based exclusively on major human allele frequency (Figure 2.4) (65). Ancestral allele state was not predictive of association to fluoxetine response.

While this study produced several encouraging results, it was also subject to some limitations. The most obvious drawback of this study is the small sample size. This contributes to wide confidence intervals and diminished power to detect associations between genotype and phenotype. For example, to detect a difference in allele frequencies of 0.2 between responders and non-responders with $\alpha = 0.05$ and $1-\beta = 0.8$ would require almost a tripling of the total sample size (66). This is a critical limitation, as it suggests a much higher likelihood that our observations may contain more false negative results than if we had a much larger sample size. We also believe that the highly characterized phenotypes used in this study helps to compensate for this limitation. Also, multiple statistical comparisons were made with the data generated from this study. However, at this point, it is unclear how to correct for multiple testing with data of this type, since the comparisons made were not independent. High levels of linkage disequilibrium and low haplotype diversity indicate that the individual loci are correlated and that using a standard Bonferroni correction would be overly conservative. Further research into this statistical problem needs to be performed to fully understand how to interpret data from association studies investigating large number of SNPs and thus these results should be considered preliminary until replicated. A further limitation may involve our choice of D' to estimate LD. Although D' can be upwardly biased with small sample sizes, it is robust to differences in allele frequencies and our sample of 96 may be adequate to capture a reasonable estimate of LD in the gene regions studied (67). A final limitation might be our focus on a binary trait, antidepressant response, as our primary outcome variable. Continuous outcome variables (such as quantitative changes in symptoms) can often provide more information than a binary trait. However, the difficulty is in selecting which one to use. Trying them all would compromise our Type I error rate significantly. We thus chose the most straightforward outcome variable for the present analyses.

In summary, we have used a number of innovative molecular, phenotypic, and statistical approaches to investigate the role of DNA variants in candidate genes for fluoxetine response and found several interesting associations. The *TPH1* and *SLC6A4* genes seem to be nominally associated with response to fluoxetine. The *HTR2A*, *MAOA* and *TPH2* genes appear to be involved in determining the specificity of response to fluoxetine. If confirmed in further studies, polymorphisms in these genes could be a useful tool for a genetically-informed psychopharmacology of depression.

2.5 References

1.   Kessler RC, McGonagle KA, Zhao S, Nelson CB, Hughes M, Eshleman S, Wittchen HU, Kendler KS. Lifetime and 12-month prevalence of DSM-III-R psychiatric disorders in the United States. Results from the National Comorbidity Survey. *Arch Gen Psychiatry* 1994; 51(1):8-19.

2.   Kessler RC, Berglund P, Demler O, Jin R, Koretz D, Merikangas KR, Rush AJ, Walters EE, Wang PS. The epidemiology of major depressive disorder: results from the National Comorbidity Survey Replication (NCS-R). *JAMA* 2003; 289(23):3095-3105.

3.   Sackeim HA. The definition and meaning of treatment-resistant depression. *J Clin Psychiatry* 2001; 62 Suppl 1610-17.

4.   Serretti A, Lilli R, Smeraldi E. Pharmacogenetics in affective disorders. *Eur J Pharmacol* 2002; 438(3):117-128.

5.   Veenstra-VanderWeele J, Anderson GM, Cook EH, Jr. Pharmacogenetics and the serotonin system: initial studies and future directions. *Eur J Pharmacol* 2000; 410(2-3):165-181.

6.   Lerer B, Macciardi F. Pharmacogenetics of antidepressant and mood-stabilizing drugs: a review of candidate-gene studies and future research directions. *Int J Neuropsychopharmacol* 2002; 5(3):255-275.

7.   Lesch K-P, Bengel D, Heils A, Sabol SZ, Greenberg BD, Petri S, Benjamin J, Müller CR, Hamer DH, Murphy DL. Association of anxiety-related traits with a polymorphism in the serotonin transporter gene regulatory region. *Science* 1996; 274(5292):1527-1531.

8.   Serretti A, Benedetti F, Zanardi R, Smeraldi E. The influence of Serotonin Transporter Promoter Polymorphism (SERTPR) and other polymorphisms of the

serotonin pathway on the efficacy of antidepressant treatments. *Prog Neuropsychopharmacol Biol Psychiatry* 2005; 29(6):1074-1084.

9.   Kim DK, Lim SW, Lee S, Sohn SE, Kim S, Hahn CG, Carroll BJ. Serotonin transporter gene polymorphism and antidepressant response. *NeuroReport* 2000; 11(1):215-219.

10.   Yu YW, Tsai SJ, Chen TJ, Lin CH, Hong CJ. Association study of the serotonin transporter promoter polymorphism and symptomatology and antidepressant response in major depressive disorders. *Mol Psychiatry* 2002; 7(10):1115-1119.

11.   Kraft JB, Peters EJ, Slager SL, Jenkins GD, Reinalda MS, McGrath PJ, Hamilton SP. Analysis of association between the serotonin transporter and antidepressant response in a large clinical sample. *Biol Psychiatry* 2006; advanced online publication.

12.   Walther DJ, Peter JU, Bashammakh S, Hortnagl H, Voits M, Fink H, Bader M. Synthesis of serotonin by a second tryptophan hydroxylase isoform. *Science* 2003; 299(5603):76.

13.   Nakamura K, Sugawara Y, Sawabe K, Ohashi A, Tsurui H, Xiu Y, Ohtsuji M, Lin QS, Nishimura H, Hasegawa H, Hirose S. Late developmental stage-specific role of tryptophan hydroxylase 1 in brain serotonin levels. *J Neurosci* 2006; 26(2):530-534.

14.   Sanchez C, Hyttel J. Comparison of the effects of antidepressants and their metabolites on reuptake of biogenic amines and on receptor binding. *Cell Mol Neurobiol* 1999; 19(4):467-489.

15.   Sargent P, Williamson DJ, Pearson G, Odontiadis J, Cowen PJ. Effect of paroxetine and nefazodone on 5-HT1A receptor sensitivity. *Psychopharmacology (Berl)* 1997; 132(3):296-302.

16.   Zanardi R, Artigas F, Moresco R, Colombo C, Messa C, Gobbo C, Smeraldi E, Fazio F. Increased 5-hydroxytryptamine-2 receptor binding in the frontal cortex of depressed patients responding to paroxetine treatment: a positron emission tomography scan study. *J Clin Psychopharmacol* 2001; 21(1):53-58.

17.   Kim SW, Park SY, Hwang O. Up-regulation of tryptophan hydroxylase expression and serotonin synthesis by sertraline. *Mol Pharmacol* 2002; 61(4):778-785.

18.   Stokes AH, Xu Y, Daunais JA, Tamir H, Gershon MD, Butkerait P, Kayser B, Altman J, Beck W, Vrana KE. p-ethynylphenylalanine: a potent inhibitor of tryptophan hydroxylase. *J Neurochem* 2000; 74(5):2067-2073.

19.   Zimmer L, Luxen A, Giacomelli F, Pujol JF. Short- and long-term effects of p-ethynylphenylalanine on brain serotonin levels. *Neurochem Res* 2002; 27(4):269-275.

20.   Yoshida K, Naito S, Takahashi H, Sato K, Ito K, Kamata M, Higuchi H, Shimizu T, Itoh K, Inoue K, Tezuka T, Suzuki T, Ohkubo T, Sugawara K, Otani K. Monoamine oxidase: A gene polymorphism, tryptophan hydroxylase gene polymorphism and antidepressant response to fluvoxamine in Japanese patients with major depressive disorder. *Prog Neuropsychopharmacol Biol Psychiatry* 2002; 26(7-8):1279-1283.

21.   Cusin C, Serretti A, Zanardi R, Lattuada E, Rossini D, Lilli R, Lorenzi C, Smeraldi E. Influence of monoamine oxidase A and serotonin receptor 2A polymorphisms in SSRI antidepressant activity. *Int J Neuropsychopharmacol* 2002; 5(1):27-35.

22.   Serretti A, Zanardi R, Rossini D, Cusin C, Lilli R, Smeraldi E. Influence of

tryptophan hydroxylase and serotonin transporter genes on fluvoxamine

antidepressant activity. *Mol Psychiatry* 2001; 6(5):586-592.

23.   Serretti A, Zanardi R, Cusin C, Rossini D, Lorenzi C, Smeraldi E. Tryptophan

hydroxylase gene associated with paroxetine antidepressant activity. *Eur*

Neuropsychopharmacol 2001; 11(5):375-380.

24.   McGrath PJ, Stewart JW, Petkova E, Quitkin FM, Amsterdam JD, Fawcett J,

Reimherr FW, Rosenbaum JF, Beasley CM, Jr. Predictors of relapse during fluoxetine

continuation or maintenance treatment of major depression. *J Clin Psychiatry* 2000;

61(7):518-524.

25.   Stewart JW, Quitkin FM, McGrath PJ, Amsterdam J, Fava M, Fawcett J,

Reimherr F, Rosenbaum J, Beasley C, Roback P. Use of pattern analysis to predict

differential relapse of remitted patients with major depression during 1 year of

treatment with fluoxetine or placebo. *Arch Gen Psychiatry* 1998; 55(4):334-343.

26.   First MB, Spitzer RL, Gibbon M, Williams JBW: Structured Clinical Interview

for DSM-IV Axis I Disorders-Patient Edition (SCID-I/P). New York, Biometrics

Department, New York State Psychiatric Institute, 1995.

27.   Quitkin FM, Rabkin JG, Ross D, Stewart JW. Identification of true drug

response to antidepressants. Use of pattern analysis. *Arch Gen Psychiatry* 1984;

41(8):782-786.

28.   McGrath PJ, Stewart JW, Quitkin FM, Chen Y, Alpert JE, Nierenberg AA,

Fava M, Cheng J, Petkova E. Predictors of relapse in a prospective study of fluoxetine

treatment of major depression. *Am J Psychiatry* 2006; 163(9):1542-1548.

29.   Quitkin FM. Placebos, drug effects, and study design: a clinician's guide. *Am J*

Psychiatry 1999; 156(6):829-836.

30.   Iyengar S, Seaman M, Deinard AS, Rosenbaum HC, Sirugo G, Castiglione CM,

Kidd JR, Kidd KK. Analyses of cross species polymerase chain reaction products to

infer the ancestral state of human polymorphisms. *DNA Seq* 1998; 8(5):317-327.

31.   Chen X, Levine L, Kwok PY. Fluorescence polarization in homogeneous

nucleic acid analysis. *Genome Res* 1999; 9(5):492-498.

32.   Hamilton SP, Slager SL, Heiman GA, Deng Z, Haghighi F, Klein DF, Hodge

SE, Weissman MM, Fyer AJ, Knowles JA. Evidence for a susceptibility locus for

panic disorder near the catechol-O-methyltransferase gene on chromosome 22. *Biol

Psychiatry* 2002; 51(7):591-601.

33.   Rozen S, Skaletsky HJ: Primer3 on the WWW for general users and for

biologist programmers., in Bioinformatics Methods and Protocols. Edited by Krawetz

S, Misener S. Totowa, NJ, Human Press, 2000, pp 365-386.

34.   Yuan X, Yamada K, Ishiyama-Shigemoto S, Koyama W, Nonaka K.

Identification of polymorphic loci in the promoter region of the serotonin 5-HT2C

receptor gene and their association with obesity and type II diabetes. *Diabetologia*

2000; 43(3):373-376.

35.   Rotondo A, Schuebel K, Bergen A, Aragon R, Virkkunen M, Linnoila M,

Goldman D, Nielsen D. Identification of four variants in the tryptophan hydroxylase

promoter and association to behavior. *Mol Psychiatry* 1999; 4(4):360-368.

36.   Hamilton SP, Slager SL, Heiman GA, Deng Z, Haghighi F, Klein DF, Hodge

SE, Weissman MM, Fyer AJ, Knowles JA. Evidence for a susceptibility locus for

panic disorder near the catechol-O-methyltransferase gene on chromosome 22. *Biol

Psychiatry* 2002; 51(7):591-601.

37.   Hamilton SP, Slager SL, Heiman GA, Haghighi F, Klein DF, Hodge SE,

Weissman MM, Fyer A.J., Knowles JA. No genetic linkage or association between a functional promoter polymorphism in the monoamine oxidase-A gene and panic disorder. *Mol Psychiatry* 2000; 5(5):465-466.

38.   Melke J, Landen M, Baghei F, Rosmond R, Holm G, Bjorntorp P, Westberg L, Hellstrand M, Eriksson E. Serotonin transporter gene polymorphisms are associated with anxiety-related personality traits in women. *Am J Med Genet* 2001; 105(5):458-463.

39.   Ihaka R, Gentleman R. R: A language for data analysis and graphics. *J Comput Graph Stat* 1996; 5(3):299-314.

40.   Freidlin B, Zheng G, Li Z, Gastwirth JL. Trend tests for case-control studies of genetic markers: power, sample size and robustness. *Hum Hered* 2002; 53(3):146-152.

41.   Sham PC, Curtis D. Monte Carlo tests for associations between disease and alleles at highly polymorphic loci. *Ann Hum Genet* 1995; 59(Pt 1):97-105.

42.   Schneider S, Roessli D, Excoffier L. Arlequin: A software for population genetics data analysis. 2000; Genetics and Biometry Lab, Dept.of Anthropology, University of Geneva, version 2.000.

43.   Ke X, Cardon LR. Efficient selective screening of haplotype tag SNPs. *Bioinformatics* 2003; 19(2):287-288.

44.   Abecasis GR, Cookson WO. GOLD--graphical overview of linkage disequilibrium. *Bioinformatics* 2000; 16(2):182-183.

45.   Bacanu SA, Devlin B, Roeder K. The Power of Genomic Control. *Am J Hum Genet* 2000; 66(6):1933-1944.

46.   Johnson GC, Esposito L, Barratt BJ, Smith AN, Heward J, Di Genova G, Ueda H, Cordell HJ, Eaves IA, Dudbridge F, Twells RC, Payne F, Hughes W, Nutland S, Stevens H, Carr P, Tuomilehto-Wolf E, Tuomilehto J, Gough SC, Clayton DG, Todd

JA. Haplotype tagging for the identification of common disease genes. *Nat Genet* 2001; 29(2):233-237.

47.   Cardon LR, Palmer LJ. Population stratification and spurious allelic association. *Lancet* 2003; 361(9357):598-604.

48.   Devlin B, Roeder K, Wasserman L. Genomic control, a new approach to genetic-based association studies. *Theor Popul Biol* 2001; 60(3):155-166.

49.   Pritchard JK, Rosenberg NA. Use of unlinked genetic markers to detect population stratification in association studies. *Am J Hum Genet* 1999; 65(1):220-228.

50.   Weinshilboum R. Inheritance and drug response. *N Engl J Med* 2003; 348(6):529-537.

51.   Pollock BG, Ferrell RE, Mulsant BH, Mazumdar S, Miller M, Sweet RA, Davis S, Kirshner MA, Houck PR, Stack JA, Reynolds CF, Kupfer DJ. Allelic variation in the serotonin transporter promoter affects onset of paroxetine treatment response in late-life depression. *Neuropsychopharmacology* 2000; 23(5):587-590.

52.   Gelernter J, Kranzler H, Coccaro EF, Siever LJ, New AS. Serotonin transporter protein gene polymorphism and personality measures in African American and European American subjects. *Am J Psychiatry* 1998; 155(10):1332-1338.

53.   Caspi A, Sugden K, Moffitt TE, Taylor A, Craig IW, Harrington H, McClay J, Mill J, Martin J, Braithwaite A, Poulton R. Influence of life stress on depression: moderation by a polymorphism in the 5-HTT gene. *Science* 2003; 301(5631):386-389.

54.   Gelernter J, Kranzler H, Cubells JF. Serotonin transporter protein (SLC6A4) allele and haplotype frequencies and linkage disequilibria in African- and European-American and Japanese populations and in alcohol-dependent subjects. *Hum Genet* 1997; 101243-246.

55.   Gabriel SB, Schaffner SF, Nguyen H, Moore JM, Roy J, Blumenstiel B, Higgins J, DeFelice M, Lochner A, Faggart M, Liu-Cordero SN, Rotimi C, Adeyemo A, Cooper R, Ward R, Lander ES, Daly MJ, Altshuler D. The structure of haplotype blocks in the human genome. *Science* 2002; 296(5576):2225-2229.

56.   Rioux JD, Daly MJ, Silverberg MS, Lindblad K, Steinhart H, Cohen Z, Delmonte T, Kocher K, Miller K, Guschwan S, Kulbokas EJ, O'Leary S, Winchester E, Dewar K, Green T, Stone V, Chow C, Cohen A, Langelier D, Lapointe G, Gaudet D, Faith J, Branco N, Bull SB, McLeod RS, Griffiths AM, Bitton A, Greenberg GR, Lander ES, Siminovitch KA, Hudson TJ. Genetic variation in the 5q31 cytokine gene cluster confers susceptibility to Crohn disease. *Nat Genet* 2001; 29(2):223-228.

57.   Martin ER, Lai EH, Gilbert JR, Rogala AR, Afshari AJ, Riley J, Finch KL, Stevens JF, Livak KJ, Slotterbeck BD, Slifer SH, Warren LL, Conneally PM, Schmechel DE, Purvis I, Pericak-Vance MA, Roses AD, Vance JM. SNPing away at complex diseases: analysis of single-nucleotide polymorphisms around APOE in Alzheimer disease. *Am J Hum Genet* 2000; 67(2):383-394.

58.   Zhang K, Calabrese P, Nordborg M, Sun F. Haplotype block structure and its applications to association studies: power and study designs. *Am J Hum Genet* 2002; 71(6):1386-1394.

59.   Bialik RJ, Ravindran AV, Bakish D, Lapierre YD. A comparison of placebo responders and nonresponders in subgroups of depressive disorder. *J Psychiatry Neurosci* 1995; 20(4):265-270.

60.   Rausch JL, Johnson ME, Fei YJ, Li JQ, Shendarkar N, Hobby HM, Ganapathy V, Leibach FH. Initial conditions of serotonin transporter kinetics and genotype: influence on SSRI treatment trial outcome. *Biol Psychiatry* 2002; 51(9):723-732.

61. Mayberg HS, Silva JA, Brannan SK, Tekell JL, Mahurin RK, McGinnis S, Jerabek PA. The functional neuroanatomy of the placebo effect. *Am J Psychiatry* 2002; 159(5):728-737.

62. Leuchter AF, Cook IA, Witte EA, Morgan M, Abrams M. Changes in brain function of depressed subjects during treatment with placebo. *Am J Psychiatry* 2002; 159(1):122-129.

63. Reich DE, Goldstein DB. Detecting association in a case-control study while correcting for population stratification. *Genet Epidemiol* 2001; 20(1):4-16.

64. Devlin B, Roeder K, Bacanu SA. Unbiased methods for population-based association studies. *Genet Epidemiol* 2001; 21(4):273-284.

65. Hacia JG, Fan JB, Ryder O, Jin L, Edgemon K, Ghandour G, Mayer RA, Sun B, Hsie L, Robbins CM, Brody LC, Wang D, Lander ES, Lipshutz R, Fodor SP, Collins FS. Determination of ancestral alleles for human single-nucleotide polymorphisms using high-density oligonucleotide arrays. *Nat Genet* 1999; 22(2):164-167.

66. Dupont WD, Plummer W.D. PS: A power and sample size program available for free on the Internet. *Controlled Clin Trials* 1997; 18(2):274-280.

67. Weiss KM, Clark AG. Linkage disequilibrium and the mapping of complex human traits. *Trends Genet* 2002; 18(1):19-24.

CHAPTER 3

SEQUENCING OF PHARMACODYNAMIC CANDIDATE GENES[*]

3.1 Introduction

In the previous chapter, I describe an indirect association study, in which I

genotyped evenly spaced, largely non-coding, publicly available SNPs (N=93) in six

serotonin genes in a well characterized sample (N=96) of depressed individuals taking

fluoxetine (2). Several variants were significantly (p<0.05) associated with fluoxetine

response and response specificity, including variants in HTR2A, TPH1, TPH2, and

MAOA. Odds ratios for these single locus associations ranged from 2-5 (rare allele

carrier relative to non-carrier). Full-length haplotypes of SNPs in these genes were

also associated with response and response specificity. These initial results prompted

the work described in this chapter, which has two main goals. The first is to follow-

up on the positive indirect association study by resequencing all exons, intron-exon

boundaries, and 5' conserved non-coding sequence of six pharmacodynamic genes in

the same depressed population taking fluoxetine. We resequenced the *HTR1A*,

HTR2A, HTR2C, TPH1, TPH2, and *MAOA* genes, but not the serotonin transporter

(*SLC6A4*) which was similarly sequenced in previous work by another graduate

student in our group (3). By undertaking this, we hope to uncover any potentially

functional variants in coding and regulatory regions that are in linkage disequilibrium

(LD) with previously associated SNPs. The second goal, which will be expanded on

in the next chapter, is to use the combined variant data set (results from previous

genotyping and current resequencing) to define the LD structure of these six genes

---

[*] Components of this work have been published (1) and are reprinted with permission. Other sections
have been submitted for publication (Peters E.J., Slager S.L., McGrath P.J., Hamilton S.P. 2007
"Sequencing and tagging SNP selection in serotonin-related candidate genes and association to
citalopram response.")

and select tagging SNPs for future studies. The high density of the 188 variants in the combined data set allows us to define the variation in these six important serotonin candidate genes, which will be useful in larger studies investigating anti-depressant response and other serotonergic psychiatric phenotypes.

While this project was ongoing, Zhang *et al.* reported on a naturally occurring, functional, Arg441His (R441H) missense variant in the human tryptophan hydroxylase 2 (*TPH2*) gene (4). The frequency of the His441 allele was higher in the 87 depressed patients (0.06) than among 219 controls samples (0.009). This association is strengthened by their *in vitro* work, which showed that this substitution reduced serotonin synthesis by approximately 80% in a heterologous expression assay in a rat cell line. We, along with our collaborators, sequenced exon 11 and genotyped a number of samples (N=2,519) of subjects with and without depression and did not detect a single His441 allele, as detailed in our letter to the journal *Neuron* and expanded on in this chapter (1).

3.2 Methods

3.2.1 Study populations. The study population consisted of 95 research subjects enrolled in an NIMH-funded protocol (Patrick J. McGrath, Columbia University, principal investigator) to assess relapse following fluoxetine discontinuation in depressed subjects who had responded to fluoxetine. The sample used in this current study is a subset of a larger population (N=96) that has been extensively described in the previous chapter as part of our study using publicly available markers (2). In searching for the R441H *TPH2* variant described by Zhang *et al.*, we also utilized the Coriell Human Variation Collection panel of 100 unrelated Caucasians and panel of 100 unrelated African Americans, as well as the STAR*D sample set which is

83

described in detail in the next chapter. Several genomic DNA (gDNA) samples were kindly provided by Marc Caron's group (Duke University) to assist in assay development; these included two Arg441 (GG) homozygote samples, a heterozygote (AG) sample, and a His441 (AA) homozygote sample. Additionally, they graciously provided samples of the DNA clone used in their lab for genotyping assay development (Figure 3.1).

3.2.2 Pharmacodynamic gene variant discovery. Patient genomic DNA was extracted from whole blood using a Puregene genomic DNA purification kit (Gentra Systems, Minneapolis, MN, USA). DNA was quantified using an ND-1000 spectrophotometer (NanoDrop Technologies, Rockland, DE, USA). PCR primers were designed to amplify all exons and ~20 bp of flanking intronic sequence of the six genes. We also sequenced 5' proximal conserved non-coding sequence (CNS) identified using mammalian global sequence alignments. For this study, we used the VISTA genome browser and searched 5 kb of DNA 5' proximal of the transcriptional start site and defined CNS as sequence that had at least 70% identity in both human-mouse and human-rat comparisons (minimum window size = 100 bp) (5). Primers were designed using Primer3 software and were manufactured by Invitrogen (Carlsbad, CA, USA) (6). Primer sequences and amplicon information are shown in Table 3.1. PCR reactions of 5 microliters (μl) containing 200 nM of the forward and reverse primers, 20 ng genomic DNA template, 50 μM dNTPs (Roche, Indianapolis, IN, USA), 1M anhydrous betaine (Acros Organics, Geel, Belgium), 50 mM KCl, 20 mM Tris-HCl (pH 8.4), 2.5 mM MgCl$_2$, and 0.25 U Platinum Taq DNA polymerase (Invitrogen, Carlsbad, CA, USA). Samples were cycled using a touchdown protocol at 94°C for 3 min, followed by seven cycles of 94°C for 30 s, 65–59°C for 30 s (decreased by 1°C intervals per cycle), and 72°C for 30 s, followed by 38 cycles of

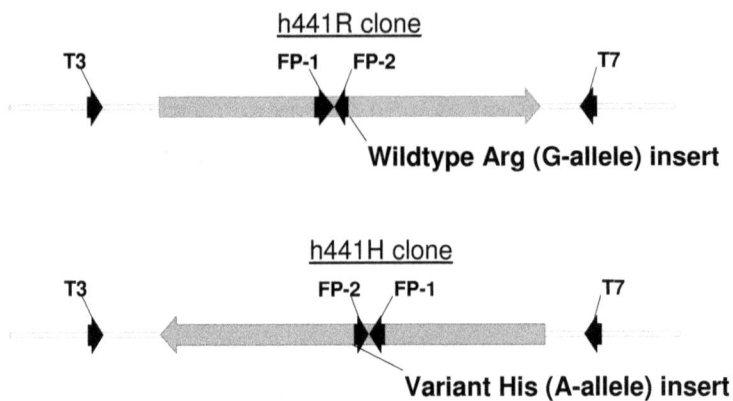

Figure 3.1. hTPH2 clone schematic. These clones were used for genotyping assay development by the Caron group, whom kindly provided them to our group. These vectors each have a 492bp insert, however, the variant His (A) insert has the opposite orientation compared to the wildtype Arg (G) insert. Also shown are the two FP probes (FP-1 and FP-2) we used to determine insert orientation.

Amplicon name	BAC	Chr.	Length	Start	Stop	Forward / Reverse primer seq
HTR1A Pro Amp 1	AC122707	5	455	63293984	63294439	CGGAGGTACCGTTTTGTTGT TCCCTCTAGCTCAGCGTCTT
HTR1A Pro Amp 2	AC122707	5	849	63293256	63294105	GGTGGTGATGTGGTGTTGTT TGGAGGCGGAGTTTATTTGT
HTR1A Amp 1	AC122707	5	649	63291642	63292291	GGCGGCTGTGTGTACAGTTT GCCCGAGAGAGGAAGACAGT
HTR1A Amp 2	AC122707	5	685	63292199	63292884	CAGAACAAGAGCCACGATGA ACCCCATCGACTACGTGAAC
HTR1A Amp 3	AC122707	5	696	63292722	63293418	CCATGATCCTTGCTAATGGTG CATTCCCTTCCTCCGAAACT
HTR2A Pro Amp 1	AL160397	13	661	46368351	46369012	CGCTCGGGAAGATAAATGTC GCCAACAGGATCCTAGCAGT
HTR2A Pro Amp 2	AL160397	13	812	46368036	46368848	GGGTGGCATATTTCTGCTG TTCTGTGACTCGCTGCATCT
HTR2A Pro Amp 3	AL160397	13	829	46369887	46370716	GGCAAGCAGGGTACAGGTAG CCCTGGACAAATTCAACCAC
HTR2A Amp 1	AL160397	13	693	46367533	46368226	GCCACCACAGTTCAGTTCTTT TAGTTTGTTTGCCCCCTGAG
HTR2A Amp 2	AL160397	13	561	46364361	46364922	GCATTCATCAGCCAGTGCTA TCTTTCCTGAAGCGAATCTGA
HTR2A Amp 3	AL136958	13	683	46307367	46308050	ATAATCAGAAAAATGTGGCATAAAA ATGAAGAAAGGGCACCACAT
HTR2A Amp 4	AL136958	13	676	46306774	46307450	GTCCATCAGCAATGAGCAAA TGCTGTCAGAACATTTTCCAAG
HTR2A Amp 5	AL136958	13	699	46306243	46306942	CACACTGAGCAAGTTTTCACCT AAGACCACACTGGAAATTCAGA
HTR2A Amp 7	AL136958	13	598	46305183	46305781	TTTGGGAGGCTGAGATGG TGAAATGAGTGAGTTTTTGGAGA
HTR2C Pro Amp 1	AC007022	X	840	113722477	113723317	CTCCGGCTCAGTCTTACAGG GAATCCTCTGATTCCCTCCA
HTR2C Pro Amp 2	AC007022	X	451	113724506	113724957	TTTGGGGAGGGGTATGCTAT TCATATGCAATCGGCAGGTA
HTR2C Amp 2	AC007022	X	493	113754293	113754786	CCCAGCCTCTATTCACGATG TCAGGTTGCATTAAAATGCTGT
HTR2C Amp 3	AC004822	X	449	113867246	113867695	TGAAGCCATGTCTACTCCAAGA GAGCAAGCTACCAAGCAAAGTTA
HTR2C Amp 4	AC004822	X	664	113871881	113872545	GTTGTTTTGCATGAGCAACG GCAACTAACTGTTCATTCATTGTTT
HTR2C Amp 5	AL590097	X	392	113988669	113989061	CACCATCATCATCCCTATAGAAAA TAGCCGCTGCAATTCTTATG
HTR2C Amp 6	AL355812	X	823	114047268	114048091	TCGATTATGCCGTGAATAGC TAAGCTCCCTCCCAGACAAA
HTR2C Amp 7	AL355812	X	672	114048032	114048704	GCCTCCTGTCAGGCAGATT GAGCAGAGCAAGAATGTAAAGTG
HTR2C Amp 8	AL355812	X	665	114048641	114049306	CAAATTCAGTGGACATTTGTTCTG GGGCCCAATTCTGTAGTCCT
HTR2C Amp 9	AL355812	X	843	114049128	114049971	TGTGCTTCACACAAAGTGAAAT TGGCAGTGTTGCAAATCAA

Table 3.1. Sequencing amplicon information.

Amplicon name	BAC	Chr.	Length	Start	Stop	Forward / Reverse primer seq
HTR2C Amp 10	AL355812	X	659	114049899	114050558	ACAAGGGCAGTGGAAGAGC TTGTTTCATACCAAACTGCACA
HTR2C Amp 11	AL355812	X	691	114050440	114051131	CAGCACATTTGTTAATGATTCTTG TCATGAGGAATTGGTGATGCT
MAOA Pro Amp 3	AL109855	X	698	43399643	43400341	GGTCTTAGCGAGAGTACTGACTCC GGGAGCTGGGCACTGAGA
MAOA Amp 1	AL109855	X	500	43400159	43400659	CCACCTCAGTGCCTGACA GGTTCCCCTACCCCTCACT
MAOA Amp 2	AL109855	X	200	43427664	43427864	GCATTTGAATGTTACGTTGCTC TCCAGTGGTGCCACTTGTAG
MAOA Amp 3	AL020990	X	369	43437307	43437676	ATTGTGCCCCAGTTCTTGAG TGTTTTCTCAAATAAAATGCTTCC
MAOA Amp 4	AL020990	X	269	43472299	43472568	AAACATGACATTCTCTGACTCCTG CCTGGGAGAAAGCAAAATCA
MAOA Amp 5	AL020990	X	830	43475376	43476206	ATTTTCCTTCCTTGGGCTTT GTGTGGCCAAGGATATGAGG
MAOA Amp 6	AL020990	X	212	43476825	43477037	ATGTGTGTATGGGTGTCTCTGAT CCAATACATCAACACAATTTGGAA
MAOA Amp 7	AL020990	X	246	43480356	43480602	AAAGGGCAGCTCTTAAAATAAACA GGTTGGTTTGTTGGAATTTTG
MAOA Amp 8	AL020990	X	247	43484814	43485061	CCCATCAGTTACTCCTTCCCTA TTATCCTCCAAGTTAAGCATATCG
MAOA Amp 9	AL020990	X	228	43486083	43486311	ACTCGCAGCATTTCAGCTTT TGCATTGAACTCTGCTTTTCC
MAOA Amp 10	AL020990	X	490	43487939	43488429	CCCACCTTCCCAAGTAACTC GGAGATGTGAGTTTTATGTTCCA
MAOA Amp 11	AL020990	X	595	43488501	43489096	TTTGTTCCTCCTTGTCAGCA CCTACTCCACCTCCACAGACA
TPH1 Pro Amp 1	AC055860	11	793	18024031	18024824	GTTGCTCTGCCTCAAGGAAT GACTTGGGTTGGACTCTGGA
TPH1 Pro Amp 2	AC055860	11	800	18023634	18024434	CGCCCGCTTCTATAAGAGAC TTTCCTGGGTTAGCAAGTTCA
TPH1 Pro Amp 3	AC055860	11	538	18023011	18023549	ATATGTTATCACTGAGGTCCATTTGT CCAACTGGTACCCTTTTCTCA
TPH1 Amp 2	AC055860	11	509	18013970	18014479	GTTTCTGGAGGATGGGATGA GCAATTTGGAGAGCTTGTGTT
TPH1 Amp 3	AC055860	11	478	18011614	18012092	AGCTAAAATTAAAACTCTCATCCAA GAGACCAAGGCAGGTGGA
TPH1 Amp 4	AC055860	11	526	18007242	18007768	TTCCCAAATATCATTTGTCAAGTA AACAGAGTTCAGCAACTCCCTTA
TPH1 Amp 5	AC055860	11	299	18004542	18004841	ACGTGTTACTTGGTGCCACT AACCCATAAGGTAGATGCCATT
TPH1 Amp 6	AC055860	11	390	18003578	18003968	TTTGATTAGTGTCCTTTGTGATCC ACTGCAACCTCCAAGCAAAG
TPH1 Amp 7	AC055860	11	296	18001898	18002194	GGGTATTTTGGGTCAGTGACTA GACATCCCAAGTATGTTCCAT
TPH1 Amp 8	AC055860	11	316	18000814	18001130	TGAGCCAATTATGGAAGTTGC TCCTTGTGGGCTTCAAATTA

Table 3.1 (con't). Sequencing amplicon information.

Amplicon name	BAC	Chr.	Length	Start	Stop	Forward / Reverse primer seq
TPH1 Amp 9	AC055860	11	398	17999453	17999851	GGGACCTCTGCAAATGTAGTGTA
						CAAGAGATGGCCCAGACCT
TPH1 Amp 10	AC055860	11	669	18025553	18026222	TGGGTAGCATGGACATTTGA
						AGGGGTGGCTCTAAGACGTT
TPH1 Amp 11	AC055860	11	680	18024938	18025618	CACTTTTGCTTGATTATTGATGGT
						TTGTGAACAACAGGACATAGAGG
TPH2 Pro Amp 1	AC090109	12	662	70616773	70617435	CTTGGCACGTTTGTTGAAAA
						TGTAAGGGTCAGCTCTAATCAGC
TPH2 Pro Amp 2	AC090109	12	576	70617608	70618184	TCAAACAAGCACATTTGGTCA
						TTGTGCATGCAAATGTGTGA
TPH2 Pro Amp 3	AC090109	12	691	70618300	70618991	TGTTCGGGAGCACAATAATTT
						GCGGAGATTGAGAGGAAGG
TPH2 Amp 1	AC090109	12	577	70618626	70619203	GGCAGGCTTGAGAGATGAGA
						GGTGAGGAGAAGATGGTCACA
TPH2 Amp 2	AC090109	12	279	70621573	70621852	GGAGGATTCTGGAACCCTAACTA
						CATAGCAGATAACAGGTTTGTACCC
TPH2 Amp 3	AC090109	12	582	70624239	70624821	GTGTGGGTACTTGGCACCTT
						AGCATTGCAGCACAGAACAT
TPH2 Amp 4	AC090109	12	494	70629416	70629910	TTAGCCTGAATTGCCACACA
						TGTGGCTCACAGGTCTCATT
TPH2 Amp 5	AC090109	12	441	70652414	70652855	TGCACAACATTAGAAGGTTAGCAT
						CTGCAACCTGTGTCCTTGG
TPH2 Amp 6	AC090109	12	296	70658921	70659217	AAATAGTAGAAGCTCCTGCTTGG
						AACAGGGCCTAAGTCATTTTCA
TPH2 Amp 7	AC090109	12	381	70674353	70674734	TCCCAGCATTGATGAACTGTA
						GGTAAATTCACCATGTTTTCTCC
TPH2 Amp 8	AC090109	12	467	70702260	70702727	CATTCAACCTAGGGAGAGAATACTG
						AAAGGCATGACCCATTTTCA
TPH2 Amp 9	AC090109	12	780	70711239	70712019	TGTGATGTCATGGAGCTTCG
						AGATGCAGTTTGGTTAAGGACA
TPH2 Amp 10	AC090109	12	692	70711917	70712609	TCCAATGGCAGATAACCACTC
						CTGCTTCAGGCAAATCACAA

Table 3.1 (con't). Sequencing amplicon information. Amplicons with "Pro" listed after the gene name amplify putative promoter region DNA, all other amplicons target exonic sequence. The BAC that the amplicon maps to is shown, as well as the length in basepairs. Chromosomal start and stop coordinates of the amplicons are listed relative to the March 2006 assembly (hg18) of the human genome.

90°C for 30 s, 58°C for 30 s, and 72°C for 30 s, with a final 10 min at 72°C. The reactions were performed on an Applied Biosystems GeneAmp PCR System 9700 (Foster City, CA, USA) using 384-well plates (MJ Research, Waltham, MA, USA). PCR products were run on a 1% agarose gel to confirm the specificity of the reaction and that product was of expected size. Unsuccessful reactions were redesigned with different primers. PCR products were prepared for sequencing by incubating product with exonuclease I (0.5 U/sample) and shrimp alkaline phosphatase (2.5 U/sample) at 37°C for 90 min and inactivating the enzymes at 95°C for 15 min. DNA sequencing of PCR product as template was performed using BigDye cycle sequencing on an ABI 3730 DNA analyzer. All amplicons in all samples (N=95) were sequenced in at least one direction, with the optimal strand choice based on sequencing both strands of a subset of these samples (N=6). Sequencing traces were analyzed for polymorphisms using Mutation Surveyor v2.4.1 (Soft Genetics, State College, PA) and confirmed by visual inspection. Variants identified on only one or two chromosomes in our population were confirmed by sequencing the opposite strand. Hardy–Weinberg equilibrium for each SNP was calculated using the Arlequin 2.0 software suite (7).

3.2.3 TPH2 Arg441His variant genotyping. In addition to the 95 depressed subjects taking fluoxetine, we sequenced 200 Coriell Human Diversity samples for *TPH2* exon 11, using the same methods described above. Furthermore, we used several different methods to genotype the control DNA sent from the Caron group, including allele specific PCR (AS-PCR), Taqman and FP-TDI. FP-TDI was performed as described in Chapter 2, and Taqman was performed as described in Chapter 4. AS-PCR was performed as described in Zhang *et al.* (4). Primer sequences and locations can be found in Figure 3.2. The RNAse P quantitative PCR assay was run in duplicate using 1 ul or 2 ul of control gDNA from the Caron group, on an ABI 7900 according to manufacturers' protocol.

3.2.4 Characterization of variable amino acids. In order to investigate whether any of the cSNPs that we uncovered may affect protein function, we tested the level of conservation for each variable amino acid position using the SIFT (Sorting Intolerant From Tolerant) program (8). This program uses protein sequence as input, and then performs an iterative psi-blast of the SWISSPROT/TrEMBL database in order to create an alignment of all available orthologous and paralogous protein sequences above a user defined cutoff for median conservation. We used a median conservation of 3.9 and dropped sequences with >95% identity in this analysis. The score for whether a particular amino acid change is predicted to be tolerated is based on the site specific conservation; a low score (e.g., <0.05) indicates that this position is highly conserved in the alignment, a higher score indicates that this position is variable.

3.2.5 Population genetic parameter estimation. We calculated two estimators of the population mutation parameter theta (θ), based on the number of segregating sites (θ_s), and the mean number of pairwise differences (π). θ_s was estimated as $(S/a_1)/B$, where S is the number of segregating sites, B is the number of nucleotides sequenced, and $a_1 = \sum_{i=1}^{n-1} \frac{1}{i}$, where n is the number of chromosomes investigated ($a_1 = 5.827$ for autosomal genes and 5.550 for X-linked genes in this study) (9). π was estimated as $(\sum_{j=1}^{S} 2p_j(1-p_j))/((1-(1/n))$ divided by the number of nucleotides sequenced, where p_j is the observed frequency of the jth SNP (10). We calculated θ_s and π for the coding

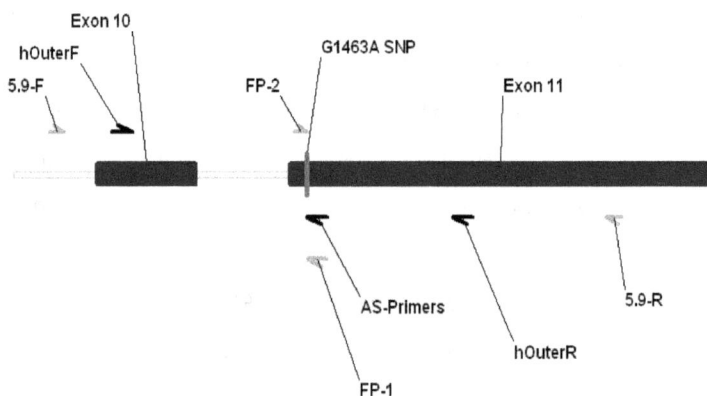

Primer Name	Sequence
hOuterF	ATGTGTGAAAGCCTTTGACCCAAAGACA
hOuterR	TGCGTTATATGACATTGACTGAACTGCT
AS-G-allele	TAGGGATTGAAGTATACTGAGAAGGCAC
AS-A-allele	TAGGGATTGAAGTATACTGAGAAGGCAT
5.9-F	TGTGATGTCATGGAGCTTCG
5.9-R	AGATGCAGTTTGGTTAAGGACA
FP-1	GGGATTGAAGTATACTGAGAAGGGA
FP-2	TTGCAAAGTCAATTACCC
Taqman-F	CTGTTTATTCTGCAGGGACTTTGC
Taqman-R	TCTGTGTGTAGGGATTGAAGTATACTGA
Taqman AlleleG (VIC)	TCAATTACCCGTCCCTTC
Taqman AlleleA (FAM)	CAATTACCCATCCCTTC

Figure 3.2. Primer location and sequences for the TPH2 Arg441His (G1463A) variant. Taqman primers and probes, which are not shown on the schematic, flank the SNP by a total of ~40 bp on each side.

regions of all genes, and calculated aggregate values for each functional gene region using the autosomal gene data. We tested for selective effects using Tajima's D statistic, which quantifies the deviation from the neutral expectation of $\theta_s = \pi$ (11). Significance of Tajima's D statistic was tested empirically by generating random samples (N=10,000) under the hypothesis of selective neutrality and population equilibrium using a coalescent simulation algorithm, as implemented in the software suite Arlequin (7).

3.2.6 Single locus association analysis. Single locus associations were tested via logistic regression using a custom script for the statistical package R v1.6.1 (12). For each SNP, three phenotypic comparisons were made based on the results from the response pattern analysis described in the sample description. The comparisons made were: (1) all responders (specific and nonspecific) vs nonresponders, (2) specific responders vs both nonspecific responders and nonresponders, and (3) specific responders vs nonspecific responders. Genotypes were coded as 0, 1, or 2 corresponding to the presence of 0, 1, or 2 copies of the rare allele, and unconditional logistic regression was used to assess the association between genotype and response phenotype. For each SNP with significant genotypic association (p<0.05), odds ratio estimates and 95% confidence intervals were computed, comparing carriers of the rare allele to non-carriers.

3.2.7 Haplotype association analysis. Haplotype analysis was performed using all common SNPs (>10% minor allele frequency, N=97) identified in this population, including 63 SNPs genotyped in the study described in the previous chapter. Haplotypes were inferred using a PL-EM algorithm, as implemented in the program TagSNPs (13). In order to limit haplotype diversity for haplotype association testing, regions of low haplotype diversity ("haplotype blocks") were chosen using the program HAPLOBLOCKFINDER (14). We defined haplotype blocks as regions in which at least 80% of chromosomes assayed were represented by 3 or less common haplotypes. Common haplotypes (>0.01 population frequency) within blocks were tested for association with antidepressant response using COCAPHASE v2.43 (15). This program uses an EM algorithm to obtain maximum likelihood estimates of haplotype frequencies and uses standard unconditional logistic regression to calculate likelihood ratio tests under a log-linear model of the probability that a haplotype belongs to the case rather than the control group.

3.3 Results

3.3.1 DNA sequencing. In order to expand on the results of an earlier indirect association study using evenly spaced publicly available SNP makers, we sequenced the coding region, intron-exon boundaries, and 5' flanking conserved non-coding sequence (CNS) of six serotonin pathway genes (*HTR1A*, *HTR2A*, *HTR2C*, *TPH1*, *TPH2*, and *MAOA*) in a subset (N=95) of the clinical population used in our previous study. This sample set consisted of subjects of primarily Caucasian descent, as identified by self-report. With this sample set, we had 85.2% power to detect autosomal (*HTR1A*, *HTR2A*, *TPH1*, and *TPH2*) gene variants at 1% MAF and 76.7% power to detect X-linked (*MAOA* and *HTR2C*) gene variants at 1% MAF. We had >99.9% power to detect variants with 5% MAF in all genes investigated. We sequenced approximately 32 kb of DNA per subject (3 Mb overall) and identified 115 variants (Table 3.2). Most of the variants identified were rare, in fact 52 of the variants were seen on only one of 190 chromosomes screened (N=144 chromosomes for X-linked *MAOA* and *HTR2C*). Two single and one two basepair insertion-deletion (indel) polymorphisms were observed; the rest of the variants were SNPs. All three indels were only seen on a single chromosome and had no entry in dbSNP build 124. We identified 60 polymorphisms that were novel and not in public databases, none of these were common in our population.

Of the 115 variants that we uncovered in these six genes, 11 of them were non-synonymous (Table 3.3). We identified four novel cSNPs, however, all of them were seen on only a single chromosome in our population and thus are not likely to be common in future studies of these genes in Caucasian individuals. We analyzed the amino acid conservation of the variants with the SIFT algorithm. Four SNPs had SIFT scores <0.05, and thus altered an evolutionarily conserved amino acid. While three of the four SNPs predicted to be intolerable changes were seen on a single chromosome in our population, a notable exception was the His452Tyr substitution in the *HTR2A* receptor which had a SIFT score of 0.02 and had a MAF of 11% in our population.

We estimated the population genetic parameters θ_s and π for each of the genes investigated (Table 3.4). Since our sequencing data is unbiased in terms of SNP selection, the comparison of these two estimates of nucleotide diversity can be used to calculate Tajima's D statistic. Tajima's D statistic can indicate whether these genes are under strong negative selective pressure (high frequency of rare variants), or under strong positive selection pressure (high frequency of common variants). Given that the entire fluoxetine sample set has major depression, indicators of strong selection in serotonergic candidate genes in this population may lend additional evidence to the serotonergic hypothesis of depression. The coding region of the *TPH1* gene had the lowest nucleotide diversity, with only two low frequency synonymous variants detected ($\pi = 2.4 \times 10^{-5}$). Tajima's D estimates for coding regions were negative for half of the genes investigated, and was significantly negative for the *HTR1A* coding

Gene	Amplicon	MAF	Position	Region	AA Change	FP?	dbSNP ID	Singleton?	Indel?	Context Sequence
HTR1A	Pro 1	0.474	-1019	CNS	-	FP	rs6295	-	-	GTAGCTTTTTAAAAA(G/C)GAAGACACACTCGGT
HTR1A	Pro 2	0.005	-117	CNS	-	-	-	Singleton	-	CCTGCTTGGGTCTCT(G/T)CATTCCCTTCCTCCG
HTR1A	3	0.005	81	NS	Ile->Val	-	rs1799921	-	-	GGCAACACTACTGGT(A/G)TCTCCGACGTGACCG
HTR1A	3	0.005	194	S	Arg->	-	-	Singleton	-	CATCGCCTTGGAGCG(C/T)TCCCTGCAGAACGTG
HTR1A	3	0.021	293	S	Val->	FP	rs6294	-	-	CGCGCTGTATCAGGT(G/A)CTCAACAAGTGGACA
HTR1A	3	0.005	506	S	Ile->	-	-	-	-	CTTCCTCATCTCTAT(C/T)CCGCCCATGCTGGGC
HTR1A	2	0.026	551	S	Pro->	-	-	-	-	AGACCGCTCGGACCC(C/T)GACGCATGCACGATT
HTR1A	2	0.005	658	NS	Arg->Leu	FP	rs1800044	Singleton	-	ATGGGCGCATATTCC(G/T)AGCTGCGCGCTTCCG
HTR1A	1	0.005	1444	3'	-	-	-	Singleton	-	TCCACGGCAGGGCCC(T/G)TTGTGCAAAGGAGAC
HTR1A	1	0.495	1528	3'	-	-	rs6449693	-	-	CATTGGCTCAGACTT(C/T)GCCTGTATCATCAGT
HTR1A	1	0.495	1555	3'	-	FP	rs878567	-	-	CAGTTTTGATCCCAG(T/C)AATTGCCTCTTCTCT
HTR2A	Pro 3	0.011	-2609	CNS	-	-	-	-	-	CACTCCCATGCCTAC(A/T)CTCCTGCAGTCCCTT
HTR2A	Pro 3	0.005	-2563	CNS	-	-	-	Singleton	-	TCATTCCTATTGATA(T/G)TCTTACTGATATTAA
HTR2A	Pro 3	0.005	-2500	CNS	-	-	-	Singleton	-	ATGTGTGTAAGTATT(T/C)GGCCCATGTCTGGCT
HTR2A	Pro 3	0.111	-2263	CNS	-	-	rs731244	-	-	GCCCCCCTCACTGCC(A/C)TGCCTGCCACCCTCC
HTR2A	Pro 3	0.437	-2225	CNS	-	-	rs731245	-	-	GAGATCTAGCCACCT(A/G)TTTCCTGGGTGGGTG
HTR2A	Pro 3	0.005	-2135	CNS	-	-	-	-	-	TGCCAGATCCCACTT(C/T)GTCTCCGGTGCTACC
HTR2A	Pro 2	0.447	-1437	CNS	-	FP	rs6311	-	-	AGTGCTGTGAGTGTC(C/T)GGCACTTCCATCCAA
HTR2A	Pro 2	0.063	-1420	CNS	-	-	rs6306	-	-	AAACAGTATGTCCTC(G/A)GAGTGCTGTGAGTGT
HTR2A	Pro 2	0.026	-1272	CNS	-	-	rs6315	-	-	GCTACATATTAATAT(T/C)GGGAAGTTTTCCTTT
HTR2A	Pro 2	0.005	-1182	CNS	-	-	rs6316	-	-	TCAGACCTCCCTCTA(T/C)GTGTATGTCATAAGC
HTR2A	Pro 1	0.005	-1007	CNS	-	-	-	Singleton	Indel	GGTTCCTCCCTCCCT(/het_insC)GTGCGGCTCGCCTCA
HTR2A	Pro 1	0.079	-783	CNS	-	FP	rs6312	-	-	ATTTGTCTTCAGGGT(C/T)CACACATGAGATACA
HTR2A	Pro 1	0.005	-559	CNS	-	-	rs6309	-	-	TCTCAGCCATTCTTA(A/G)GCTGAATTGCCACAG
HTR2A	1	0.011	73	NS	Thr->Asn	-	rs1805055	-	-	TTACTGTAGAGCCTG(G/T)TGTCATCATTTAATT
HTR2A	1	0.005	92	S	Asp->	-	-	Singleton	-	TTCTCCGGAGTTAAA(G/A)TCATTACTGTAGAGC
HTR2A	1	0.447	101	S	Ser->	FP	rs6313	-	-	AGTGTTAGCTTCTCC(G/A)GAGTTAAAGTCATTA
HTR2A	1	0.005	217	NS	Glu->Gly	-	-	Singleton	-	GCAGACCAGTTTTTT(T/C)CCTGGAGATGAAGTA
HTR2A	2	0.300	3260	Intron	-	-	rs2296973	-	-	CTCCTGGAGCACATG(T/G)ATCCCTATCCTATGA
HTR2A	2	0.016	3419	S	Asp->	FP	rs6305	-	-	GATGGCGACGTAGCG(G/A)TCCAGCGAGATGGCG
HTR2A	2	0.016	3492	NS	Ile->Val	FP	rs6304	-	-	TGGTCCAAACAGCAA(T/C)GATTTTCAGAAATGC
HTR2A	2	0.005	3602	Intron	-	-	-	Singleton	-	GATTGAGGATGTCAG(G/A)TTTCAGTACAACAAA
HTR2A	4	0.005	60893	S	Thr->	-	-	Singleton	-	GGCCAAAGCCGGTAT(T/A)GTGTTCACTAAAATT
HTR2A	4	0.105	61008	NS	His->Tyr	FP	rs6314	-	-	AAGCCTCTTCAGAAT(G/A)CTGCTTTCCTAGAGC
HTR2A	4	0.005	61037	S	Ser->	-	-	Singleton	-	TTCATTCACTCCGTC(G/A)CTATTGTCTTTAGAA
HTR2A	5	0.179	61191	3' UTR	-	FP	rs3125	-	-	ATAAAATGAGGCATA(C/G)AGATATGATCGTTGG
HTR2A	5	0.200	61472	3' UTR	-	-	rs3803189	-	-	AAAATTTTCACTATT(T/G)ATAGCTATTTTTATT
HTR2A	6	0.005	62101	3' UTR	-	-	-	Singleton	-	ATAAATAGTATAAAC(C/T)GATGGATCTGAAAGC
HTR2A	7	0.011	62550	3'	-	-	-	-	-	AGTTTAGTCATTTTC(T/C)TTTTTTCTTTCTTTT
HTR2A	7	0.005	62580	3'	-	-	-	Singleton	-	CTGTATATATTTTTT(G/T)ACTAAGACCATTTCA
HTR2A	7	0.116	62612	3'	-	-	rs11148016	-	-	GGAAATAAGTTGAAA(T/G)GATTCTAAAAATAAG
HTR2C	Pro 1	0.007	-144652	CNS	-	-	-	Singleton	-	TTCTGGCGGGACTCG(T/A)ATTTATTTTGTCAGA
HTR2C	Pro 1	0.153	-144529	CNS	-	-	rs3795182	-	-	ACAGTAATTTATAAA(T/C)ATGGAAGAGAAAACG
HTR2C	1	0.153	-142827	CNS	-	FP	rs3813929	-	-	TCTTGGGCCAAAAGC(G/A)GGATGAGGGGAGGAG
HTR2C	1	0.389	-142765	5' UTR	-	FP	rs518147	-	-	GAAGGAAGCGTCCTC(C/G)GCAAGCACCAGAGCG
HTR2C	1	0.007	-142619	5' UTR	-	-	-	Singleton	-	GCGACGACTCCGACG(A/T)CAACGATGTACAGAC
HTR2C	2	0.021	-113028	5' UTR	-	-	-	-	-	TTTTTGAAGGATGGC(G/A)TCAGTTGGCCTATGT
HTR2C	2	0.021	-112989	Intron	-	-	-	-	-	AAGAGTCTTGAGGCA(C/T)GCTTATGTGTATACT
HTR2C	2	0.007	-112853	Intron	-	-	-	Singleton	-	TTTACCAATTACATA(A/G)TATTCTTTTTCAAAC
HTR2C	3	0.007	-277	Intron	-	-	-	Singleton	-	TTATTTATCATCGCA(A/G)ATTTTTAAAAATTTTC
HTR2C	3	0.007	-176	Intron	-	-	-	Singleton	-	TGCACTTAATGGTGA(T/A)AAGAAACAGTTATTA
HTR2C	3	0.229	63	Intron	-	FP	rs2248440	-	-	GCAAAGTTATCTTTT(C/T)ACTAAAATAATAAGT
HTR2C	4	0.222	4388	NS	Cys->Ser	FP	rs6318	-	-	CTCACAGAAATATCA(C/G)ATTGCCAAACCAATA
HTR2C	5	0.181	121190	Intron	-	-	rs5946005	-	-	GAGAAGACAAGAACA(C/T)GTCATCCAAATTGTA
HTR2C	6	0.007	180119	NS	Arg->Gln	-	-	Singleton	-	ACCAGAACGCACGCC(G/A)AAGAAAGAAGAAGGA
HTR2C	7	0.007	181019	3' UTR	-	-	-	Singleton	-	ATGACAGTGGTTATA(T/G)TTCAACCACACCTAA
HTR2C	8	0.056	181359	3' UTR	-	-	rs1801412	-	-	ACTTCTTAAGGACAG(T/G)GTTCAAATTCTGATT
HTR2C	8	0.007	181432	3' UTR	-	-	-	Singleton	-	TTAGTAAATTCCTAA(T/C)TCTATGATTAAACTG
HTR2C	8	0.014	181443	3' UTR	-	-	-	-	-	CTAATTCTATGATTA(A/C)ACTGGGAAATGAGAT
HTR2C	9	0.007	182160	3' UTR	-	-	-	-	-	GAATTCATGATGCTA(G/A)TATTCTTACGCTTGACA
HTR2C	10	0.007	182360	3' UTR	-	-	-	Singleton	-	CTCTATTTGATTTGC(A/G)ACACTGCCAAACATC
HTR2C	10	0.007	182365	3' UTR	-	-	-	Singleton	-	TTTGATTTGCAACAC(T/G)GCCAAACATCAGTCA
HTR2C	11	0.028	183284	3'	-	-	rs5987830	-	-	ATTAAATGTTGGCTA(A/C)TATGTCACATGTCTT

Table 3.2. Pharmacodynamic gene variants uncovered during resequencing.

Gene	Amplicon	MAF	Position	Region	AA Change	FP?	dbSNP ID	Singleton?	Indel?	Context Sequence
TPH1	10	0.337	-7228	CNS	-	FP	rs6486405	-	-	GAGTATTTTATAGTT(T/G)TCATTGTAGAGATCT
TPH1	10	0.347	-7113	CNS	-	FP	rs6486404	-	-	ATTGGCATACAGAAA(C/T)GCTATTGATTTTTGT
TPH1	10	0.011	-7067	CNS	-	-	rs11024455	-	-	CCTGCAACATTAGTG(A/C)ATTATTTAATCAGTT
TPH1	10	0.005	-6951	CNS	-	-	-	Singleton	Indel	TCCAGTTTGGATGCC(C/het_del)TTTATTTCTTCTCTT
TPH1	10	0.011	-6873	CNS	-	-	rs11024454	-	-	GGTGAAATTGGGCAT(C/A)CTTATCGTGTTCCAG
TPH1	10	0.005	-6867	CNS	-	-	-	Singleton	-	ATTGGGCATCCTTAT(C/T)GTGTTCCAGATCTAC
TPH1	11	0.005	-6616	CNS	-	-	-	Singleton	-	TGTACCTCATAGAAG(C/T)ATTATACAGATAAAA
TPH1	11	0.358	-6574	CNS	-	-	rs4537731	-	-	AGAAAAGCTGTAAAG(A/G)TCCTGAGCTTTAAAG
TPH1	11	0.005	-6501	CNS	-	-	-	Singleton	-	ACAAATCACTAATAC(C/T)TGCATGAAACTCAAA
TPH1	11	0.011	-6398	CNS	-	-	rs12273833	-	-	AAGGCAAAACTGTGG(A/G)GACAGAAATCAGATC
TPH1	12	0.332	-5855	CNS	-	FP	rs7130929	-	-	CCAGAAGCACAGAGA(G/T)GTGTGGGAGGTGGGG
TPH1	12	0.011	-5776	CNS	-	-	-	-	-	GCAGGTCATTGTGTC(G/C)ATAATAGGCGTTATC
TPH1	Pro 2	0.005	-5277	CNS	-	-	-	Singleton	Indel	GGAGAAAAGACACTT(TT/het_del)TGAGTGCCTCCTGTG
TPH1	Pro 2	0.332	-4873	CNS	-	-	rs6486403	-	-	GTCAGTTAAGAGTCC(G/A)TGTGAAACTCAACCTT
TPH1	Pro 3	0.358	-4353	CNS	-	-	rs7122118	-	-	TGTGCTTCCTAGATC(C/A)GGTAAATATAAATTA
TPH1	1	0.200	-174	CNS	-	-	rs10488682	-	-	TTTTGGTCTCACTAG(A/T)TTCTTGCAAAGCTTA
TPH1	3	0.453	7531	Intron	-	-	rs10832874	-	-	AGTCTTGCTCTGCTG(T/C)CCAGACTGGAGTGCA
TPH1	4	0.005	11318	Intron	-	-	-	Singleton	-	AGAATAAATTGTGTT(C/T)ATTTGGTAAGTAGAA
TPH1	4	0.011	11466	S	Gln->	-	-	-	-	GGGAACCGTATTCCA(A/G)GAGCTCAACAAACTC
TPH1	5	0.016	14284	Intron	-	-	-	-	-	GCCGTAAGTACTTCT(A/G)TTTCAGCCAGGAATT
TPH1	6	0.453	15053	Intron	-	FP	rs1799913	-	-	CAAACTTGTACCTCT(C/A)TTTCAGAGATACCTG
TPH1	8	0.005	17898	S	Leu->	-	-	Singleton	-	CAAACAGGAATGTCT(T/C)ATCACAACTTTTCAA
TPH1	9	0.005	19795	Intron	-	-	-	Singleton	-	GTCATCCAGGAACAT(T/C)TGAGCATCAATTCGG
TPH1	9	0.005	19800	Intron	-	-	-	Singleton	-	CCAGGAACATTTGAG(C/T)ATCAATTCGGAGGTC
TPH2	Pro 1	0.021	-1971	CNS	-	-	-	-	-	GGTTCAGCTTCCCA(T/G)GACTGCAAAGCCTTT
TPH2	Pro 1	0.084	-1913	CNS	-	-	rs11178996	-	-	TAATTTTTTGTTGCC(A/G)TTGTTTTCCAACTTA
TPH2	Pro 1	0.005	-1782	CNS	-	-	-	Singleton	-	TTATAAATAAATTAC(T/G)TTTAATATGTTTTTT
TPH2	Pro 1	0.021	-1666	CNS	-	-	-	-	-	CATTAGCTACTATTA(T/C)TGTCATTAGTTCATT
TPH2	Pro 2	0.005	-1178	CNS	-	-	-	Singleton	-	TAACGCACAGATCTC(G/T)TATATTTAAGTAGCA
TPH2	Pro 2	0.005	-888	CNS	-	-	-	Singleton	-	GCCCTTTTATGAAAG(G/T)CATTACACATATATA
TPH2	Pro 3	0.084	-614	CNS	-	-	rs11178997	-	-	TTTGATCATTACACA(T/A)TGTACGCTTGTGTCA
TPH2	1	0.011	-52	5' UTR	-	-	rs11178998	-	-	TCCGCCAGCGCTGCT(A/G)CTGCCCCTCTAGTAC
TPH2	2	0.005	2613	NS	Ser->Tyr	-	-	Singleton	-	TAAATAAACCTAACT(C/A)TGGCAAAAATGACGA
TPH2	4	0.026	10520	Intron	-	-	rs11179003	-	-	AATTGAACACTACC(C/T)ACCACAGTGATTTTC
TPH2	5	0.458	33419	Intron	-	-	rs7963720	-	-	TGGGATCCTTTCAGA(C/T)GCTCATGTGCTCCAC
TPH2	6	0.432	40095	S	Pro->	-	rs7305115	-	-	TCCCCTCTACACCC(A/G)GAACCGTGAGTACCT
TPH2	7	0.189	55607	Intron	-	-	rs1007023	-	-	CAACTTAAAACCAGT(G/T)CTATTTATGTCCATT
TPH2	7	0.026	55657	Intron	-	-	-	-	-	CAGGATTATTGACTA(T/C)GAGTTATAGGTAAAT
TPH2	8	0.347	83468	S	Ala->	-	rs4290270	-	-	AGGGCAACTGCGGGC(A/T)TATGGAGCAGGACTC
TPH2	9	0.016	92483	Intron	-	-	-	-	-	CTTTTATCTATCCCT(C/T)GTACCAATGAGGGTT
TPH2	10	0.116	93187	3' UTR	-	-	-	-	-	CATCACAATAACAAA(G/A)GTTCAATATTCTATT
TPH2	10	0.005	93218	3' UTR	-	-	-	Singleton	-	TCAAAAATTGTTGAG(G/A)TAACACAGCAGTTGG
MAOA	Pro 3	0.007	-579	CNS	-	-	-	Singleton	-	GGGAGCTCCTATACC(C/T)AATGACCTTTCGCAA
MAOA	Pro 3	0.007	-537	CNS	-	-	-	Singleton	-	AGCACCTCCTACACC(C/T)AGTAACACCCCCGAG
MAOA	4	0.007	53505	Intron	-	-	-	Singleton	-	ACAGGAGTCAGAGAA(T/A)GTCATGTTTTTTACAA
MAOA	5	0.007	56904	Intron	-	-	-	Singleton	-	CAACCAAGGCTGGTA(A/G)TTTGGAAGACTGAGG
MAOA	6	0.306	57177	S	Arg->	FP	rs6323	-	-	AGCTCCCATTGGAAG(C/A)CGCTGAATTAACTGG
MAOA	10	0.035	69450	Intron	-	-	-	-	-	GAGGCTGTATAGTTT(C/T)TACAGATTCAAGGCC
MAOA	10	0.306	69532	S	Asp->	-	rs1801291	-	-	TTCTTGTACCCAGAT(A/G)TCTTTCTCGGTCACC
MAOA	10	0.007	69533	NS	Ile->Val	-	-	Singleton	-	GTTCTTGTACCCAGA(T/C)ATCTTTCTCGGTCAC
MAOA	11	0.007	69876	NS	Lys->Arg	-	rs1800466	Singleton	-	GGCAGGAGCTTGTAT(T/C)TGTACAGCACAAACC

Table 3.2 (con't). Pharmacodynamic gene variants discovered during resequencing. Displayed are all 115 variants discovered during resequencing, as well as the amplicon, minor allele frequency (MAF), and position from the translational start site. Also shown are the region (CNS – conserved non-coding region, S – synonymous change, NS – non-synonymous change, 5' – 5' proximal region, 3' – 3' proximal region, UTR – untranslated region) and amino acid change if applicable. SNPs also assayed via FP-TDI are indicated as "FP", and dbSNP IDs are shown for known SNPs (dbSNP build 124). SNPs with alleles seen on a single chromosome are designated with "Singleton" and insertion/deletion polymorphism are designated with as "Indel". DNA sequence flanking the variants is also shown.

Gene	AA position	dbSNP rs#	No. of chromsomes	No. of seqs used for alignment	SIFT score
HTR1A	I28V	1799921	1	11	0.32
HTR1A	R220L	1800044	1	13	**0.02**
HTR2A	T25N	1805055	2	7	0.18
HTR2A	E73G	N/A	1	7	**0.00**
HTR2A	I197V	6304	3	13	0.76
HTR2A	H452Y	6314	20	13	**0.02**
HTR2C	C23S	6318	32	5	0.10
HTR2C	R288Q	N/A	1	16	0.36
TPH2	S41Y	N/A	1	12	0.91
MAOA	I471V	N/A	1	18	**0.04**
MAOA	K520R	1800466	1	17	0.10

Table 3.3. SIFT scores for the 11 non-synonymous SNPs. The SIFT algorithm was used to predict *in silico* the function of the amino acid altering SNPs. A median conservation of 3.9 was used and we dropped sequences with >95% identity for this analysis. Where applicable, dbSNP IDs are shown. Also shown are the number of chromosomes that the minor allele was observed (N=190). A SIFT score of <0.05 indicates a lack of conservation and thus potentially altered protein function. Only one common variant, the well-known His452Tyr SNP in HTR2A, was predicted to have altered function using this method.

	DNA sequenced (kb)	$\theta_s \times 10^4$	$\pi \times 10^4$	Number of SNPs uncovered	Number of novel SNPs
5' Conserved non-coding	11.1	7.7	7.1	51 (30)	24 (5)
Intronic	6.6	5.8	4.9	22 (13)	14 (5)
Untranslated region	6.0	4.6	2.7	16 (8)	11 (3)
Amino acid coding	8.2	5.0	3.8	26 (12)	11 (1)
Synonymous				15 (8)	7 (1)
Non-synonymous				11 (4)	4 (0)
Total	31.9			115 (63)	60 (14)

Table 3.4a

Gene	$\theta_s \times 10^4$	$\pi \times 10^4$	Tajima's D	$P(D_{obs} > D_{sim})$
HTR1A	8.12	1.06	-1.78	0.02
HTR2A	11.14	5.85	-1.09	-
HTR2C	2.62	2.63	0.00	-
TPH1	2.57	0.24	-1.25	-
TPH2	3.50	6.51	1.39	-
MAOA	5.25	6.42	0.42	-
Average	5.53 +/- 3.45	3.79 +/- 2.83	-0.38 +/- 1.19	-

Table 3.4b

Table 3.4. Population genetic parameters for the pharmacodynamic genes.
a) Variant identification summary for the six genes. θ_s and π are shown per nucleotide sequenced. Values in parentheses are for a subset of SNPs in which the minor allele was seen in at least 2 out of 190 chromosomes (i.e., non-singletons). Novel SNPs are defined as variants that were not in dbSNP build 124.
b) Population genetic parameter estimates for coding regions of the six candidate genes. θ_s and π are shown per nucleotide sequenced. Overall parameter estimates are listed as mean +/- SD for the six genes. Significance of Tajima's D departure from neutrality is also shown if nominally significant (p<0.05).

region. While a negative Tajima's D can be caused by negative selection pressure, the estimates for these genes are within the range of values previously reported for other genomic regions and consistent with a recent expansion of the human population (16;17). Nucleotide diversity (π) was highest in the CNS ($\pi = 7.1 \times 10^{-4}$) and lowest in the protein coding (3.8×10^{-4}) and untranslated regions (2.7×10^{-4}) of these genes.

Our resequencing effort identified 20 SNPs that were initially genotyped using fluorescence polarization detection of template-directed dye-terminator incorporation (FP-TDI) in our previous study. We found 2 out of 1900 matched calls were inconsistent between genotyping using FP-TDI and sequencing, yielding a reproducibility across assays of 99.89%. This value is reassuring given the substantial effect genotyping errors can have on haplotype inference (18).

3.3.2 TPH2 Arg441His variant. A highly publicized report of the functional Arg441His TPH2 variant by Zhang *et al.* was of substantial interest to us, since we had not observed this variant in our fluoxetine population (N=95). We thus sequenced an additional 200 unrelated individuals (Coriell Diversity Panel) for exon 11 and did not observe a single His441 allele. The STAR*D sample set (N=1,941) was also genotyped for this variant by our colleagues, and not a single instance of the His441 allele was found. Thus, we genotyped 2,036 DNA samples from patients with major depression for a total of 4,072 alleles and did not see this non-synonymous variant. Using our data and assuming a binomial distribution, we can rule out the His441 allele as being as frequent as 0.06 in depressed individuals (Table 3.5). Based on a threshold probability of 0.01, the maximum allele frequency in major depression is 0.001.

In order to validate our genotyping assays, we received four genomic DNAs from the Caron group; two homozygous Arg (GG) samples, a heterozygous (AG) sample, and a homozygous His (AA) sample. Several experiments were performed on these control samples, and the results are summarized in Table 3.6. We initially performed the ARMS ASPCR method that is described in Zhang *et al.*, and all the genotypes were concordant with the expected genotypes. Next, a Taqman allelic discrimination assay for the Arg441His variant was run on the controls, and again the results were concordant with expected genotypes. We then ran an FP-TDI assay specific for the Arg441His variant on the controls. For the initial PCR step of the FP-TDI, I used the sequencing primers for exon 11 (5.9-F and 5.9-R). The genotypes were concordant with expected for all samples *except* the His homozygote sample (AA), which was genotyped by FP-TDI as GG. Note that the primers for this assay lie outside the cloned 492 bp insert region (Figure 3.2). The control samples were then amplified using the exon 11 sequencing primers and products were sequenced. Genotyping results were again concordant with expected for all samples *except* the His homozygote sample (AA), which again was genotyped as GG. We then amplified the control samples with the primers for the ASPCR (hOuterF and hOuterR, which are internal to the cloned insert region), and sequenced the products. Using these primers, results were concordant with expected genotypes for all control samples. At this point, contamination of genomic DNA with clone seemed like a possibility. In order to quantify the amount of genomic DNA in these control samples, an RNAse P quantitative PCR assay was performed. All samples had expected amounts of signal from the RNAse P probe, *expect* for the His homozygote sample (AA), which had no detectable product. So as to verify that the discordant genotyping results were due to clone contamination in the sample, four PCRs were performed (Table 3.6,

His allele frequency	Probability of not detecting allele
0.06	7×10^{-116}
0.03	3×10^{-58}
0.01	7×10^{-20}
0.005	3×10^{-10}
0.0025	2×10^{-5}
0.001	0.01
0.0005	0.11

Table 3.5. Probability of not detecting the variant TPH2 His441 allele in 2,036 depressed subjects. Several putative His allele population frequencies are shown, with the corresponding probability of not detecting the variant allele in our population, assuming a binomial distribution.

Exp	Method	Primer F	Primer R	Internal primer(s)	Control gDNA samples				Clone DNA samples	
					GG-1	GG-2	AG	AA	Arg (G)	His (A)
1	ASPCR	hOuterF	hOuterR	A or G AS-primer	GG	GG	AG	AA		
2	Taqman	Taqman-F	Taqman-R	Taqman Allele A + G	GG	GG	AG	AA		
3	FP-TDI	5.9-F	5.9-R	FP-1	GG	GG	AG	**GG**		
4	Sequencing	5.9-F	5.9-R		GG	GG	AG	**GG**		
5	Sequencing	hOuterF	hOuterR		GG	GG	AG	AA		
6	RNAse P qPCR									
7	PCR	T7	FP-1		+	+	+	-	+	-
8	PCR	T7	FP-2		-	-	-	+	-	+
9	PCR	T3	FP-1		-	-	-	+	-	+
10	PCR	T3	FP-2		+	+	+	-	+	-

Table 3.6. Results of experiments with the TPH2 His441Arg control samples. Genotyping results using each method are shown, with the expected genotype shown in the first row of the table. Primer sequences and positions are shown in Figure 3.2. For the RNAse P qPCR method, a + or – indicates the presence or absence, respectively, of detectable genomic DNA in the sample. For the PCR methods, a + or – indicates the presence or absence, respectively, of a specific band of the expected size, as shown in Figure 3.3.

experiments 7-10), using universal cloning primers T3 and T7, and primers FP-1 and FP-2, which are internal to the clone insert and face in opposite directions (Figure 3.1). The two clones, His441 and Arg441 have their insert in the opposite directions, allowing us to differentiate between them. The results of these PCR experiments are shown in Figure 3.3. This gel confirms that the AA control, which was supposed to contain genomic DNA representing the AA homozygote, actually contained the His441 clone, as it produced the specified band using T7 and FP-2 primers or T3 and FP-1 primers. The very small amount of genomic DNA (based on the RNAse P assay) in the AA control sample appeared to actually be homozygous GG.

3.3.3 Single locus association analysis. Variants identified during resequencing were tested for association to fluoxetine response or response specificity. Three phenotypic comparisons were made: (1) responders (N=76) vs. non-responders (N=19), (2) specific responders (N=56) vs. non-specific and non-responders (N=39), and (3) specific responders vs. non-specific responders (N=20). Genotypic association was tested using logistic regression. Given the low minor allele frequency of the coding region variants identified (80% had a MAF <0.10), our power to detect association of these variants was

limited in this sample. For instance, for medium risk alleles (e.g., OR=2.5), we had greater than 80% power to detect association of variants with >0.10 MAF (Figure 3.4). Four SNPs in the promoter region of *TPH1* showed nominally significant association to categorical response to fluoxetine (Table 3.7). These SNPs have extensive LD and occur in conserved mammalian sequence 5' proximal of the *TPH1* gene. Two coding region SNPs in the *HTR2A* gene were associated with the specificity of response (specific vs. non-specific), including the evolutionarily conserved His452Tyr substitution. Two synonymous SNPs in the *MAOA* gene were

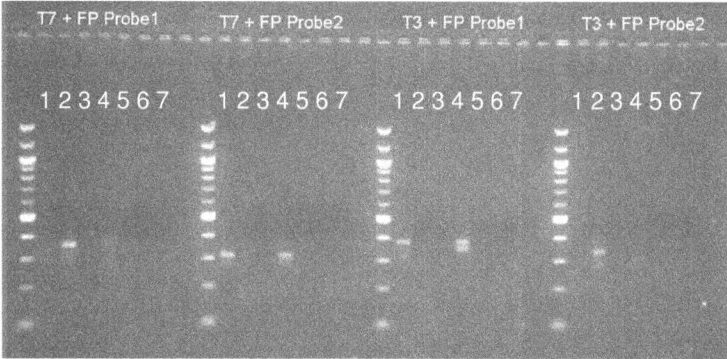

Figure 3.3. Results of PCR experiments on TPH2 Arg441His control samples. Shown are the PCR products on a 2% agarose gel, with a 100 bp ladder in the first lane of each primer combination, which is listed at the top of the gel. Lane 1: clone His (A), lane 2: clone Arg (G), lane 3: Control AG gDNA, lane 4: Control AA gDNA, lane 5: Control GG-1 gDNA, lane 6: Control GG-2 gDNA, lane 7: H2O control.

also associated with response specificity. Six of these eight associated variants were also genotyped in our previous work (2).

3.3.4 Haplotype analysis. Levels of LD varied across the genes sequenced, with *HTR1A, HTR2C, TPH1* and *MAOA* exhibiting strong LD and *TPH2* and *HTR2A* showing much lower levels of LD. In order to take advantage of all the information available on these genes, we combined the genotype data from our previous study and the current sequencing data for haplotype analysis. In our previous work, we genotyped approximately 8-10 SNPs per gene region. Genotyped SNPs were largely non-coding, with average spacing of 7.6 kb (median, 2.7 kb). The combined data set (N=188 unique SNPs) included 97 common SNPs (>10% MAF), consisting of 63 from our previous genotyping work, 19 from the current sequencing effort, and 15 that were assayed in both studies. Levels of LD may be overestimated for genomic regions when only coding region variants are included in the analysis due to the low density and minor allele frequency of these variants. This is illustrated by the results for *HTR2A*, in which we had genotype information for 15 common SNPs across the gene region, which yielded 25 inferred common haplotypes (data not shown). As expected, the addition of non-coding SNPs increased the haplotype diversity for this gene region when compared to a recent coding region centered screening in a Caucasian population of similar size (20). Full length haplotypes using all common SNPs were inferred for each gene using the EM algorithm. All of the common SNPs in *HTR1A, TPH1* and *MAOA* had strong LD and thus limited haplotype diversity and were tested for association to response using the likelihood ratio test procedure in COCAPHASE (Table 3.8). The other genes had moderate to weak LD, which made full gene length haplotype testing problematic due to the uncertainty associated with

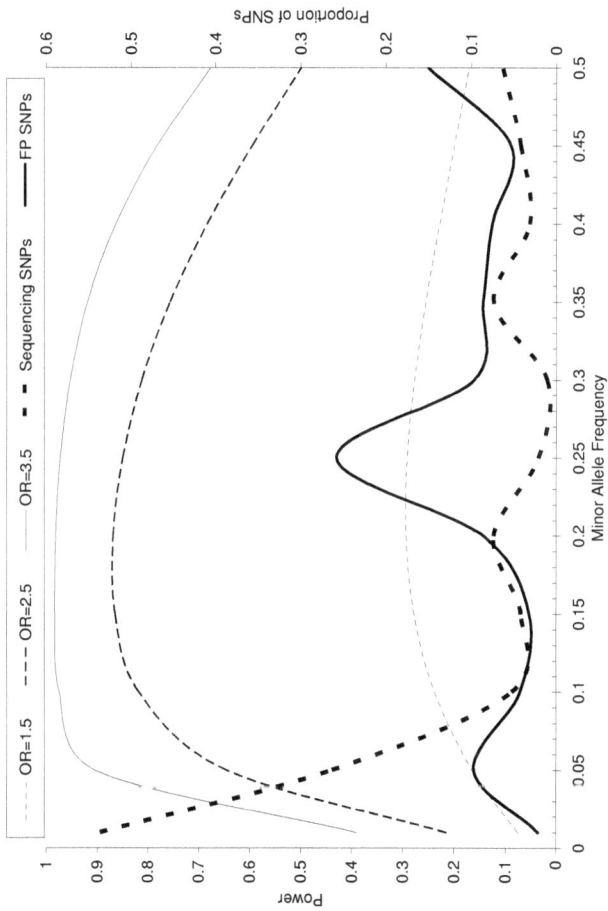

Figure 3.4

Figure 3.4. Power to detect association to categorical response in fluoxetine sample (N=95). On the left y-axis is the power $(1-\beta)$ of detecting an association at the various minor allele frequencies shown on the x-axis. Three different effect sizes (dominant ORs) are shown, indicated by the lighter lines. Power was calculated using the method of Purcell et al. (19). The right y-axis shows the proportion of SNPs at each minor allele frequency (binned in 0.02 intervals). The variants uncovered during resequencing (dark dashed line) and the variants assayed in our previous study via FP-TDI are also shown (dark solid line).

		FP?	SNP type	Response vs. Non-response				Specific response vs. Non-specific response			
				p-value	OR	Lower	Upper	p-value	OR	Lower	Upper
HTR2A											
90473	SH51	Y	NS	-				0.02	0.30	0.08	1.15
90290	SH53	Y	3' UTR	-				0.03	0.27	0.08	0.87
TPH1											
71715	SH102	Y	CNS	0.02	0.41	0.11	1.11	-			
71830	SH103	Y	CNS	0.04	0.43	0.13	1.35	-			
73088	SH112	Y	CNS	0.02	0.41	0.11	1.09	-			
74070	SH115	N	CNS	0.02	0.41	0.11	1.09	-			
MAOA											
74459	SH182	Y	S	-				0.05	0.27	0.08	0.90
62104	SH186	N	S	-				0.05	0.32	0.12	0.92

Table 3.7. Variants nominally associated (p<0.05) with response to fluoxetine. Gene name is displayed as well as SNP position. Variants genotyped via FP-TDI in our previous study (described in Chapter 2) are designated with a "Y". Odds ratios (OR) shown are calculated for variant carrier vs. non-carrier, and 95% lower and upper confidence intervals are also shown.

the inference of rare haplotypes. Gene regions were therefore partitioned into blocks of low haplotype diversity using the 0.8 chromosome coverage criteria of HAPLOBLOCKFINDER. Block size varied by gene region, with an average size of 70 kb (median = 23 kb) and an average of 1.5 blocks per gene investigated (Table 3.8). Average block size was larger than reported in previous studies on random genomic regions using Caucasian samples, which was due to the large blocks observed in the X-linked genes *MAOA* and *HTR2C* (21).

Haplotypes were constructed within blocks and tested for association to fluoxetine response (Table 3.8). A block of six SNPs in 3' end of the *HTR2A* gene was associated with response in our second phenotypic comparison, specific response versus all other responses (global p = 0.05), as well as in our third comparison, specific responders versus non-specific responders (global p = 0.01). Haplotypes of the *MAOA* gene region, which was contained in a single block, were nominally associated to response specificity in our third comparison (global p = 0.05).

3.4 Discussion

In this study, we sought to expand on the results of our previous indirect association study, which utilized evenly spaced, publicly available SNP markers in a well phenotyped patient population taking fluoxetine. Since most of the SNPs used in our previous indirect association study were intronic and non-coding, we wanted to identify putative functional SNPs associated with antidepressant response by resequencing all exons, intron-exon boundaries, and 5' conserved non-coding sequence (CNS) in this patient population. We uncovered 60 novel SNPs during resequencing, none of which were common (>10% MAF). We identified four novel non-synonymous SNPs, however these were all seen on only a single chromosome in

Gene	Block no.	Block size (kb)	SNPs/Block	Response vs. non-response	Specific vs. all others	Specific vs. non specific
HTR1A	1	7.7	8	-	-	-
TPH1	1	26.7	22	-	-	-
TPH2	1	64.9	14	-	-	-
TPH2	2	21.1	5	-	-	-
HTR2A	1	21.7	5	-	-	-
HTR2A	2	23.4	4	-	-	-
HTR2A	3	14.4	6	-	0.04	0.01
HTR2C	1	367.4	26	-	-	-
MAOA	1	81.3	7	-	-	0.04
	Average	69.8	10.8			
	Median	23.4	7			

Table 3.8. Haplotype block distribution and association results. Size of haplotype blocks and number of SNPs within each block are shown. Within-block haplotype distributions with global p-values <0.05 are shown for each phenotypic comparison, as tested in COCAPHASE.

our study population. This indicates that public databases such as dbSNP contain the majority of common cSNPs, and that further cSNP (or tagSNP) discovery efforts may be unnecessary for these genes. The database of SNPs has expanded considerably since this work was performed, and the lack of additional common variants in these genes supports this contention. We found two exonic substitutions (His452Tyr and a 3' UTR SNP) in the *HTR2A* gene and two linked synonymous SNPs in the *MAOA* gene that were associated with response specificity. The association of response subtype with the His452Tyr substitution in the *HTR2A* gene is strengthened by the evolutionary conservation seen at this genomic location and the fact that several studies have suggested that this polymorphism has altered function *in vitro* (22;23).

While most Mendelian disorders studied to date have been shown to be caused by non-synonymous coding variants or splicing variants, there is evidence that this may not be true for common, complex genetic disorders (24). Several reports have shown substantial differences in allelic expression across the human genome, and variation in regulatory DNA is a likely candidate for complex genetic phenotypes (25;26). Unfortunately, identification of regulatory DNA elements is not as straightforward as identifying protein coding sequence. We used comparative genomics in order to identify potentially functional 5' regulatory DNA sequence (CNS), and then sequenced these CNS elements in order to uncover any variants. The nucleotide diversity parameters π and θ were higher for CNS than any other region investigated, indicating that this gene region harbors substantial variation. Furthermore, much of this variation has not been investigated as we found more novel variation in CNS than in coding regions, which is where most previous variant screens have focused. By uncovering this variation, we were able to define the haplotype block structure in putative regulatory regions of these genes. In our association testing, we found four linked SNPs in the 5' CNS of the *TPH1* gene that displayed significant single locus association to categorical antidepressant response. Additionally, these SNPs have been shown to affect transcription of the *TPH1* gene *in vitro* (27).

While *in silico* methods such as comparative genomics can help to identify potentially functional elements in the genome, certain functional elements may be missed due to lack of conservation across species. This is especially true if primate-specific functional elements are present, as mammalian alignments (i.e., human and mouse, rat, or dog) might not show conservation (28). Additionally, we did not sequence the entire intronic region of these genes or CNS located outside of 5 kb upstream of the transcriptions state site, and thus may have missed functional SNPs that affect splicing or gene regulation. This may explain why we failed to find putatively functional SNPs in the coding region and 5' CNS of the *TPH2* gene, where we previously had seen an association using non-coding SNPs (2). In our population, the *TPH2* gene region contained only one non-synonymous SNP (S41Y), and this variant was seen on a single chromosome in our screen.

One limitation of this study is the small sample size of our population (N=95), which limited our power to detect association of low to medium risk alleles with antidepressant response (Figure 3.4). As most of the protein altering variants we uncovered by resequencing were extremely rare, they will require further testing in larger, perhaps family-based, clinical populations. Our limited statistical power to detect association also precluded us from performing analysis of joint association (interaction effects) between pairs of SNPs or haplotypes in these serotonergic genes and antidepressant response.

In order to expand on a previous indirect association study of antidepressant response, we sequenced the coding regions, intron-exon boundaries and 5' CNS of six serotonergic candidate genes in order to identify any potentially functional SNPs. We found four SNPs in the 5' CNS region of TPH1 that were associated with categorical response, and found the previously described His452Tyr variant and two synonymous SNPs in the *MAOA* gene to be associated with response subtype. The majority (6 of 8) of these variants were assayed in our previous work using publicly available markers. While the His452Tyr and 5' TPH1 variants have been shown to affect protein function and expression *in vitro*, further association studies in larger clinical populations will be required to determine if these variants influence patient response to antidepressants.

Given that several other groups (29-31) besides our own (1) have published letters stating they have not observed the His441 allele in unrelated sample sets, along with the fact that we were able to detect clone contamination in their control genomic DNA samples, it seems unlikely that this allele exists an any appreciable frequency in outbred human populations. It should be noted that the control His/Arg heterozygote gDNA did appear to be uncontaminated and real. However, based on our genotyping of 2,036 subjects with major depression and never observing the allele (even as a heterozygote), the maximum allele frequency of this variant is 0.001, far from the 0.06 reported in Zhang *et al.* (Table 3.5). A check of Hardy-Weinberg equilibrium on the data reported by Zhang *et al.* also points to possible genotyping problems. They report having found six heterozygotes and three homozygous His samples in their depression cohort of 87 patients. They also report on two heterozygotes and one homozygous His sample in their cohort of 219 control patients. Both the depressed cohort (χ^2=19.5, df=1, p<3.7x10^{-10}) and the control cohort (χ^2=53.5, df=1, p<1.2x10^{-}

[36]) had genotype distributions displaying an abundance of His homozygotes, several more than would be expected based on the observed minor allele frequency and Hardy-Weinberg equilibrium. Thus, it appears this variant does not contribute to the genetic risk of major depression in outbred populations.

3.5 References

1.   Zhou Z, Peters EJ, Hamilton SP, McMahon F, Thomas C, McGrath PJ, Rush J, Trivedi MH, Charney DS, Roy A. Response to Loss-of-function mutation in Tryptophan Hydroxylase-2 identified in unipolar major depression. Neuron 45, 11-16. *Neuron* 2005; 48(5):702-703.

2.   Peters EJ, Slager SL, McGrath PJ, Knowles JA, Hamilton SP. Investigation of serotonin-related genes in antidepressant response. *Mol Psychiatry* 2004; 9(9):879-889.

3.   Kraft JB, Slager SL, McGrath PJ, Hamilton SP. Sequence analysis of the serotonin transporter and associations with antidepressant response. *Biol Psychiatry* 2005; 58(5):374-381.

4.   Zhang X, Gainetdinov RR, Beaulieu JM, Sotnikova TD, Burch LH, Williams RB, Schwartz DA, Krishnan KR, Caron MG. Loss-of-function mutation in Tryptophan Hydroxylase-2 identified in unipolar major depression. *Neuron* 2005; 45(1):11-16.

5.   Couronne O, Poliakov A, Bray N, Ishkhanov T, Ryaboy D, Rubin E, Pachter L, Dubchak I. Strategies and tools for whole-genome alignments. *Genome Res* 2003; 13(1):73-80.

6.   Rozen S, Skaletsky HJ: Primer3 on the WWW for general users and for biologist programmers., in Bioinformatics Methods and Protocols. Edited by Krawetz S, Misener S. Totowa, NJ, Human Press, 2000, pp 365-386.

7.   Schneider S, Roessli D, Excoffier L. Arlequin: A software for population genetics data analysis. 2000; Genetics and Biometry Lab, Dept.of Anthropology, University of Geneva, version 2.000.

8.   Ng PC, Henikoff S. SIFT: Predicting amino acid changes that affect protein function. *Nucleic Acids Res* 2003; 31(13):3812-3814.

9.   Watterson GA. On the number of segregating sites in genetical models without recombination. *Theor Popul Biol* 1975; 7(2):256-276.

10.   Tajima F. Evolutionary relationship of DNA sequences in finite populations. *Genetics* 1983; 105(2):437-460.

11.   Tajima F. Statistical method for testing the neutral mutation hypothesis by DNA polymorphism. *Genetics* 1989; 123(3):585-595.

12.   Ihaka R, Gentleman R. R: A Language for Data Analysis and Graphics. *J Comput Graph Stat* 1996; 5(3):299-314.

13.   Stram DO, Haiman CA, Hirschhorn JN, Altshuler D, Kolonel LN, Henderson BE, Pike MC. Choosing haplotype-tagging SNPS based on unphased genotype data using a preliminary sample of unrelated subjects with an example from the Multiethnic Cohort Study. *Hum Hered* 2003; 55(1):27-36.

14.   Zhang K, Jin L. HaploBlockFinder: haplotype block analyses. *Bioinformatics* 2003; 19(10):1300-1301.

15.   Dudbridge F. Pedigree disequilibrium tests for multilocus haplotypes. *Genet Epidemiol* 2003; 25(2):115-121.

16.   Stephens JC, Schneider JA, Tanguay DA, Choi J, Acharya T, Stanley SE, Jiang R, Messer CJ, Chew A, Han JH, Duan J, Carr JL, Lee MS, Koshy B, Kumar AM, Zhang G, Newell WR, Windemuth A, Xu C, Kalbfleisch TS, Shaner SL, Arnold K, Schulz V, Drysdale CM, Nandabalan K, Judson RS, Ruano G, Vovis GF. Haplotype variation and linkage disequilibrium in 313 human genes. *Science* 2001; 293(5529):489-493.

17. Cargill M, Altshuler D, Ireland J, Sklar P, Ardlie K, Patil N, Lane CR, Lim EP,

Kalayanaraman N, Nemesh J, Ziaugra L, Friedland L, Rolfe A, Warrington J,

Lipshutz R, Daley GQ, Lander ES. Characterization of single-nucleotide

polymorphisms in coding regions of human genes. *Nat Genet* 1999; 22(3):231-238.

18. Kirk KM, Cardon LR. The impact of genotyping error on haplotype

reconstruction and frequency estimation. *Eur J Hum Genet* 2002; 10(10):616-622.

19. Purcell S, Cherny SS, Sham PC. Genetic Power Calculator: design of linkage

and association genetic mapping studies of complex traits. *Bioinformatics* 2003;

19(1):149-150.

20. Glatt CE, Tampilic M, Christie C, DeYoung J, Freimer NB. Re-screening

serotonin receptors for genetic variants identifies population and molecular genetic

complexity. *Am J Med Genet B Neuropsychiatr Genet* 2004; 124(1):92-100.

21. Patil N, Berno AJ, Hinds DA, Barrett WA, Doshi JM, Hacker CR, Kautzer CR,

Lee DH, Marjoribanks C, McDonough DP, Nguyen BT, Norris MC, Sheehan JB,

Shen N, Stern D, Stokowski RP, Thomas DJ, Trulson MO, Vyas KR, Frazer KA,

Fodor SP, Cox DR. Blocks of limited haplotype diversity revealed by high-resolution

scanning of human chromosome 21. *Science* 2001; 294(5547):1719-1723.

22. Ozaki N, Manji H, Lubierman V, Lu SJ, Lappalainen J, Rosenthal NE,

Goldman D. A naturally occurring amino acid substitution of the human serotonin 5-

HT2A receptor influences amplitude and timing of intracellular calcium mobilization.

J Neurochem 1997; 68(5):2186-2193.

23. Hazelwood LA, Sanders-Bush E. His452Tyr polymorphism in the human 5-

HT2A receptor destabilizes the signaling conformation. *Mol Pharmacol* 2004;

66(5):1293-1300.

24.   Thomas PD, Kejariwal A. Coding single-nucleotide polymorphisms associated with complex vs. Mendelian disease: evolutionary evidence for differences in molecular effects. *Proc Natl Acad Sci U S A* 2004; 101(43):15398-15403.

25.   Yan H, Yuan W, Velculescu VE, Vogelstein B, Kinzler KW. Allelic variation in human gene expression. *Science* 2002; 297(5584):1143.

26.   Morley M, Molony CM, Weber TM, Devlin JL, Ewens KG, Spielman RS, Cheung VG. Genetic analysis of genome-wide variation in human gene expression. *Nature* 2004; 430(7001):743-747.

27.   Sun HS, Fann CS, Lane HY, Chang YT, Chang CJ, Liu YL, Cheng AT. A functional polymorphism in the promoter region of the tryptophan hydroxylase gene is associated with alcohol dependence in one aboriginal group in Taiwan. *Alcohol Clin Exp Res* 2005; 29(1):1-7.

28.   Boffelli D, McAuliffe J, Ovcharenko D, Lewis KD, Ovcharenko I, Pachter L, Rubin EM. Phylogenetic shadowing of primate sequences to find functional regions of the human genome. *Science* 2003; 299(5611):1391-1394.

29.   Glatt CE, Carlson E, Taylor TR, Risch N, Reus VI, Schaefer CA. Response to Loss-of-Function Mutation in Tryptophan Hydroxylase-2 Identified in Unipolar Major Depression. Neuron 45, 11-16. *Neuron* 2005; 48(5):704-705.

30.   Van Den Bogaert A, De Zutter S, Heyrman L, Mendlewicz J, Adolfsson R, Van Broeckhoven C, Del-Favero J. Response to Loss-of-Function Mutation in Tryptophan Hydroxylase-2 Identified in Unipolar Major Depression. Neuron 45, 11-16. *Neuron* 2005; 48(5):704.

31.   Garriock HA, Allen JJB, Delgado P, Nahaz Z, Kling MA, Carpenter L, Burke M, Burke W, Schwartz T, Marangell LB, Husain M, Erickson RP, Moreno FA. Lack

of association of TPH2 exon XI polymorphisms with major depression and treatment

resistance. *Mol Psychiatry* 2005; 10(11):976-977.

CHAPTER 4

PHARMACODYNAMIC CANIDATE GENE TAGGING SNP SELECTION AND

ASSOCIATION OF TAGGING SNPS TO CITALOPRAM RESPONSE[*]

4.1 Introduction

The genotype data from our previous indirect association study (Chapter 2)

combined with the genotype data from our sequencing effort (Chapter 3) provided

dense marker coverage within these pharmacodynamic serotonin candidate genes

from which we could chose tagging SNPs. Here I describe our criteria and

performance assessment of tagging SNPs (tagSNPs), as well as our exploration of the

role of common variation in these candidate genes on antidepressant response in a

large clinical population taking the SSRI citalopram. For this purpose, we genotyped

a subset of patients (N=1,953) from the Sequenced Treatment Alternatives to Relieve

Depression (STAR*D) study, which is a prospective, multi-center, randomized

clinical trial involving 4,041 depressed outpatients in both primary and specialty care

settings (1). The overall goal of the STAR*D trial was to define what subsequent

treatment strategies, in what order or sequence, and in what combination prove most

efficacious and tolerable to patients whom have failed to respond to an initial trial

with the SSRI citalopram. STAR*D clinical findings suggest that patients who fail

initial treatment with citalopram can respond to other antidepressants (including other

SSRIs) and treatments (2), however their odds of responding decrease as more

treatments are needed (3).

In this report, we focus on five pharmacodynamic candidate genes (*HTR1A*,

HTR2A, *TPH1*, *TPH2* and *MAOA*); the *HTR2C* gene was not investigated due to lack

[*] This work has been submitted for publication (Peters E.J., Slager S.L., McGrath P.J., Hamilton S.P.
2007 "Sequencing and tagging SNP selection in serotonin-related candidate genes and association to
citalopram response.")

of any association to fluoxetine in our previous work (4). While not the focus of the work reported here, we also interrogated tagging SNPs in the serotonin transporter (*SLC6A4*) in the STAR*D population, which were not associated to citalopram response or response specificity (5). We also report on the comparison of tagSNP selection methods. In response to the substantial levels of linkage disequilibrium (LD) in the human genome and the high density SNP marker information being generated, several tagSNP selection methods have been developed to reduce redundancy in downstream genotyping and retain the genetic diversity. Some of these methods focus on using tagSNPs as proxies for untyped SNPs and thus exploit pairwise SNP LD (6). Other methods attempt to tag multimarker haplotypes, with no formal regard for pairwise SNP LD (7-9). It is unclear which method is superior, but this will likely depend on study design and resources as well as local patterns of LD. Here we use our high density SNP data to test the performance of tagSNPs selected using pairwise LD in reconstructing underlying haplotypes. This is an important comparison as we are interested in testing for haplotypic associations using haplotypes inferred from tagSNP genotypes.

4.2 Methods

4.2.1 STAR*D sample set. Of the 4,041 subjects, DNA was obtained from 1,953 subjects as part of the NIMH Human Genetics Initiative. The design of STAR*D was to enroll adults experiencing a major depressive episode who exhibited neither an inadequate response nor intolerance to an adequate trial of any of the STAR*D protocol treatments during the current episode. The overall aim of STAR*D (P.I., A. John Rush, NIMH Contract N01-MH-90003) was to prospectively determine which of a number of treatments are beneficial for subjects experiencing an unsatisfactory clinical outcome following treatment with citalopram. Since the STAR*D design trial

has been described extensively we shall only briefly summarize it here (1;10;11). In

order to make the findings as generalizable as possible, STAR*D utilized broad

inclusion criteria and enrolled a diverse population, including good minority

representation. Diagnoses were made using the Psychiatric Diagnostic Screening

Questionnaire, while depressive symptoms were assessed with the 16-item Quick

Inventory of Depressive Symptomatology collected at clinic visits (Self-Report

[QIDS-SR] version) (12). The QIDS-SR is highly correlated with the 17-item

Hamilton Rating Scale for Depression (HRSD17), and scores can be converted readily

between the two instruments (12). Subjects meeting criteria and providing consent

were administered citalopram as the initial treatment. The protocol encouraged 12

weeks of treatment with vigorous dosing of open-label citalopram (20-60 mg/day).

The sub-sample of 1,953 participants who consented to provide DNA samples was

61.8% female and 38.2% male, and with ethnic proportions of 78.1% Caucasians,

16.1% African-Americans, 3.5% multi-racial, 1.1% Asian, 1.2% Pacific

Islander/Native American, and 0.1% unspecified. Further, 14.0% of the sample

reported being Hispanic, and 43.5% of the sample came from primary care clinics,

with the remaining 56.5% coming from specialty clinics. At the time of this report,

we have received DNA from 1,914 participants (98%). Baseline demographic and

clinical data on these 1,914 subjects are presented in Table 4.1.

Access to the DNA samples and clinical data was approved by the STAR*D

Ancillary Studies Committee, and clinical data was obtained from the Data

Coordinating Center of STAR*D. Approval to carry out the work described here was

obtained by the Committee on Human Research at the University of California, San

Francisco.

4.2.2 STAR*D response phenotypic definitions. We define five inter-related response phenotype definitions of response to citalopram. The first two are responders and non-responders: responders are subjects who had at least 42 days of treatment and whose QIDS-SR on their final clinical visit shows ≥50% reduction in score; the remaining subjects, who had at least 42 days of treatment, were then considered non-responders. The ≥50% reduction in symptom severity on the HRSD17 is the conventional definition of response in clinical trials. We used the QIDS-SR score to estimate severity since all subjects had this rating and it correlates highly with the HRSD17 scores (12). We required this 42 day (or six week) threshold to ensure an adequate exposure to citalopram and to enhance the power to find associations between genotype and response by reducing potential heterogeneity. Using this threshold, we found no statistical difference in the average total dosage of citalopram between those who were on the trial for at least 42 days (average total dosage = 29.9 mg) and those who were not (average total dosage = 30.4 mg). The 254 subjects with < 42 days of treatment were excluded from analysis. The third phenotype definition is remission. Remission was defined as a QIDS-SR score ≤5, which closely corresponds to the conventional definition of a HSRD score of ≤7 (12). The final two phenotypes are based on our attempt to further reduce heterogeneity by attempting to separate placebo response from true drug response in antidepressant trials (13). Some response to antidepressant medication is a placebo response, which we posit may have either no genetic determinant or a different underlying genetic mechanism than "true" drug response. Thus, it is of interest to limit our definition of response to true pharmacologic response rather than placebo response. For these phenotypes, a "specific" pattern of response was defined by persistence, or the maintenance of response for the remainder of the study once it was attained. Previous

Baseline Variable	Total subjects in Analysis (N=1,914)	Subjects classified as Responders (N=991)	Subjects classified as Non-Responders (N=669)	p value	Subjects classified as Specific Responders (N=679)	Subjects classified as Non-Specific Responders (N=187)	Subjects Classified as Remitters (N=826)
Number in Race / Ethnicity (%)							
Caucasian	1,501 (78.4)	799 (80.6)	509 (76.1)	0.06	559 (82.3)	146 (78.1)	679 (82.2)
African American	299 (15.6)	130 (13.1)	121 (18.1)		77 (11.3)	28 (15.0)	100 (12.1)
Other (Multi-racial)	68 (3.6)	36 (3.6)	23 (3.4)		23 (3.4)	9 (4.8)	25 (3.0)
Asian	21 (1.1)	15 (1.5)	5 (0.7)		12 (1.8)	2 (1.1)	13 (1.6)
Pacific Islander/Native American	24 (1.2)	11 (1.1)	11 (1.6)		8 (1.2)	2 (1.1)	9 (1.1)
Unspecified	1 (0.1)	0	0				
Number of Hispanic (%)	269 (14.1)	122 (12.3)	102 (15.2)	0.09	82 (12.1)	25 (13.4)	96 (11.6)
Number of Females (%)	1,179 (61.6)	621 (62.7)	404 (60.4)	0.35	424 (62.4)	126 (67.4)	518 (62.7)
Mean Age in Years (SD)	42.6 (13.4)	42.2 (13.4)	43.0 (13.4)	0.11	41.7 (13.3)	43.4 (14.0)	42.0 (13.7)
Mean Years of Schooling (SD)	13.6 (3.3)	14.1 (3.3)	13.2 (3.1)	<0.001	14.2 (3.3)	13.9 (3.3)	14.2 (3.3)
Marital Status							
Married	819 (42.8)	435 (43.9)	290 (43.3)	0.27	301 (44.3)	76 (40.6)	377 (45.6)
Never Married	536 (28.0)	278 (28.1)	185 (27.7)		190 (28.0)	53 (28.3)	239 (28.9)
Divorced	483 (25.2)	249 (25.1)	162 (24.2)		169 (24.9)	52 (27.8)	189 (22.9)
Widowed	76 (4.0)	29 (2.9)	32 (4.8)		19 (2.8)	6 (3.2)	21 (2.5)
Clinical Characteristics							
Age at first MDE (SD)	26.1 (14.9)	26.2 (14.4)	25.6 (14.9)	0.19	26.4 (14.6)	24.8 (13.7)	26.4 (14.5)
Months in current MDE (SD)	25.0 (53.9)	21.6 (45.8)	31.7 (65.8)	<0.001	20.4 (45.5)	24.6 (51.5)	21.3 (45.9)
Index Length 24+ Months (%)	487 (25.4)	230 (23.2)	203 (30.3)	0.001	142 (20.9)	53 (28.3)	187 (22.6)
Presence of Recurrent Depression (%)	1,347 (70.4)	701 (70.7)	469 (70.1)	0.71	481 (70.8)	130 (70.0)	574 (69.5)
Presence of Family History of Depression (%)	1,037 (54.2)	557 (56.2)	346 (51.7)	0.09	382 (56.3)	103 (55.1)	466 (56.4)
Baseline QIDS (SD)	16.4 (3.4)	16.2 (3.3)	16.6 (3.4)	0.008	16.2 (3.3)	16.1 (3.1)	15.8 (3.3)
Years Since 1st MDE (SD)	16.6 (13.9)	16.0 (13.8)	17.5 (14.0)	0.018	15.4 (13.8)	18.6 (14.6)	15.7 (13.8)

Table 4.1. Baseline demographic and clinical characteristics of the STAR*D sample. Data shown are for the subset of DNA samples received at the time of this report (N=1,914). Tests of differences between responders and non-responders, using chi-square for categorical data and t-tests for continuous data, are presented in the column labeled "p-value".

studies considered "specific" patterns to be further characterized by delayed response, i.e., after the first two weeks (14;15). We were unable to employ this criterion because the STAR*D study design did not include ratings before week two. We defined persistent responders as those subjects who had a sustained response at all consecutive visits following the first visit with response, as measured by ≥50% reduction in QIDS-SR scores. Those whose response occurred only at the last visit were removed from the analysis. In contrast, "non-specific" responders were those subjects who did not maintain their response following the first visit with a response. Note that "specific" and "non-specific" responders are a subset of responders (as defined by the response phenotype above). Moreover, because visits were at least two weeks apart, we assumed that intervening weeks were characterized by the response defined by the previous visit. We compared "specific" responders to nonresponders, allowing us to test the hypothesis that the "specific" response to citalopram represented a more genetically homogenous group of persons taking citalopram. We also compared "specific" responders to "non-specific" responders to test whether there are genetic differences between "true drug" responders and "placebo" responders, as suggested in our previous work (4). Table 4.1 presents the demographic and clinical characteristics of our phenotype groups.

4.2.3 Tagging SNP selection. All Caucasian samples in our population taking fluoxetine (N=75) were used in tagSNP selection, regardless of response phenotype. We used the method of Carlson et al ("ldselect.pl"), which is based on pairwise LD between SNP markers and does not require haplotype block-like structure (16). We ran this algorithm to group SNPs into high LD "bins", which contain SNPs with a minimum pairwise r^2 of 0.80. A single tagSNP from each "bin" was then chosen to represent that group of SNPs in future studies. We were also interested in testing for haplotype specific effects in the study, thus we wanted to explore how accurately the

tagSNPs chosen using a pairwise r^2 threshold could reconstruct the underlying

haplotypes. In order to limit haplotype diversity and facilitate haplotype inference,

haplotype blocks were chosen using the program HAPLOBLOCKFINDER (17). We

defined haplotype blocks as regions in which at least 80% of chromosomes assayed

were represented by three or less common haplotypes. Within each haplotype block,

we then employed two haplotype tagging approaches. We used the method of Stram

et al ("TagSNPs"), which selects haplotype tagging SNPs in order to optimize R_h^2,

which is the squared correlation between estimates of the number of copies of a

particular haplotype h (inferred using only the tagSNPs) and the true number of

copies of haplotype h carried by a subject (inferred using the entire SNP set),

averaging over all possible genotype data under an assumption of Hardy-Weinberg

equilibrium (8). We also selected haplotype tagging SNPs using the pattern

recognition approach of Ke et $al.$, which does not account for the uncertainty of

inferring haplotypes for genotypic data (9). Using these three sets of tagging SNPs,

we then calculated the minimum R_h^2 for all common (>1%) haplotypes within each

haplotype block in order to asses how well these sets predict the underlying haplotype

structure.

4.2.4 DNA amplification. PCR reactions of 5 microliters (μl) containing 200 nM of

the forward and reverse primers, 10 ng genomic DNA template, 50 μM dNTPs

(Roche, Indianapolis, IN, USA), 1M anhydrous betaine (Acros Organics, Geel,

Belgium), 50 mM KCl, 20 mM Tris-HCl (pH 8.4), 2.5 mM MgCl$_2$, and 0.25 U

Platinum Taq DNA polymerase (Invitrogen, Carlsbad, CA, USA). Samples were

cycled using a touchdown protocol at 94°C for 3 minutes, followed by seven cycles of

94°C for 30 seconds, 65–59°C for 30 seconds (decreased by 1°C intervals per cycle), and 72°C for 30 seconds, followed by 38 cycles of 90°C for 30 seconds, 58°C for 30

seconds, and 72°C for 30 seconds, with a final 10 minutes at 72°C. The reactions

were performed on an Applied Biosystems GeneAmp PCR System 9700 (Foster City,

CA, USA) using 384-well plates (MJ Research, Waltham, MA, USA).

4.2.5 Tagging SNP genotyping using FP-TDI. Genotyping of tagSNPs was

performed using either fluorescence polarization detection of template-directed dye-

terminator incorporation (FP-TDI) or 5' exonuclease fluorescence assays (TaqMan)

(Table 4.2). For tagSNPs genotyped by FP-TDI, following PCR the excess primers,

deoxynucleotides, and pyrophosphate in the PCR reaction were degraded by adding

0.1μl of 10X PCR Clean-Up Reagent, containing a mixture of shrimp alkaline

phosphatase and exonuclease I (PerkinElmer, Wellesley, MA, USA), 0.1μl of

inorganic pyrophosphatase (Roche Applied Science, Indianapolis, IN, USA), and 0.8

μl of PCR Clean-Up Dilution Buffer to each 5 μl PCR reaction (PerkinElmer,

Wellesley, MA, USA). The mixture was then incubated at 37°C for 60 minutes,

followed by inactivation for 15 minutes at 80°C. The final step was the addition of a

4 μl solution containing a final concentration of 0.5 μM TDI probe, 1 μl of 10X TDI

Reaction Buffer, 0.5 μl of AcycloTerminator Mix (containing R110 and TAMRA-

labeled AcycloTerminators, corresponding to the polymorphic base), and 0.025 μl of

AcycloPol DNA polymerase (PerkinElmer). This mixture was cycled at 95°C for 2

minutes, followed by 25 cycles of 94°C for 15 seconds and 55°C for 30 seconds.

Following template-directed incorporation, fluorescence polarization was read using a

VICTOR2 1420 Multilabel Counter (PerkinElmer), and genotypes were scored using

custom software.

Gene	SNP	Assay method	Common name	Also captures
HTR1A	rs6295	FP-TDI	C-1019G	rs6449693, rs878567, rs749099, rs1423691, rs970453
HTR1A	rs1364043	C__1393788_10		rs749098
HTR2A	rs731245	FP-TDI		
HTR2A	rs6313	C__3042197_1_	T102C	rs6311 (A-1438G)
HTR2A	rs2296973	FP-TDI		-
HTR2A	rs927544	FP-TDI		-
HTR2A	rs666693	FP-TDI		-
HTR2A	rs2770296	FP-TDI		-
HTR2A	rs2246127	FP-TDI		-
HTR2A	rs1923884	C__11696916_10		-
HTR2A	rs1923882	FP-TDI		-
HTR2A	rs6314	FP-TDI	His452Tyr	rs3803189
HTR2A	rs3125	FP-TDI		rs6486405, rs6486404, rs4537731, rs6486403, rs7122118
TPH1	rs7130929	FP-TDI		rs6486405, rs6486404, rs4537731, rs6486403, rs7122118
TPH1	rs623580	FP-TDI		-
TPH1	rs684302	FP-TDI		rs1799913 (A779C), rs1800532 (A218C), rs2056246, rs1607395, rs2237907, rs10832874, rs652458, rs685249, rs211107
TPH1	rs211105	FP-TDI		rs10488682, rs172423
TPH1	rs211102	FP-TDI		-
TPH1	rs2108977	FP-TDI		-
TPH2	rs2129575	FP-TDI		-
TPH2	rs2171363	C__15836061_10		rs79637220, rs7305115
TPH2	rs1007023	C__8872308_10		rs1386488, rs1843809, rs1386492, rs1843812, rs1487281, rs1386497
TPH2	rs1487278	Custom Taqman		rs1386491, rs1487284
TPH2	rs1487276	FP-TDI		-
TPH2	rs1386487	Custom Taqman		rs4290270
TPH2	rs17110747	Custom Taqman		-
TPH2	rs1872824	FP-TDI		-
MAOA	rs1465108	C__11407441_10		rs2310820, rs1465107, rs6323, rs979606, rs979605, rs1801291

Table 4.2

128

Table 4.2. Tagging SNPs assayed in the STAR*D population. Listed are the 28 tagSNPs chosen from our genotype data in the fluoxetine population (N=75 Caucasians), using the method of Carlson *et al.*(section 4.3.1) (1). One SNP (rs2246127) was removed from the analysis after genotyping due to HWE violations. SNPs assayed via FP-TDI are designated as "FP-TDI"; details on these assays can be found in Chapter 1. SNPs interrogated using the Taqman assay indicate their Applied Biosystems assay ID (C...), assays that were custom designed by Applied Biosystems are designated "Custom Taqman". Also shown are the dbSNP IDs of the additional SNPs that are in high LD ($r^2>0.8$) with the assayed SNPs in the Caucasian subset of the fluoxetine sample.

4.2.6 Tagging SNP genotyping using 5' exonuclease fluorescence assay. For tagSNPs genotyped using 5' exonuclease fluorescence (Taqman) assays (Table 4.2), 5 μl reactions containing 10 ng of dried genomic DNA template, 2.5 μl of Universal Taqman PCR Master Mix (Applied Biosystems), 0.085 μl of 20X Taqman assay probe (Applied Biosystems), and 2.42 μl of sterile H_2O were cycled at 95°C for 10 minutes, followed by 40 cycles of 92°C for 15 seconds and 60°C for 1 minute. Reaction fluorescence was read and genotypes were scored on an ABI 7900HT Sequence Detection System (Applied Biosystems).

4.2.7 Statistical analysis. The frequency distributions of demographic and clinical variables were examined in the combined sample and by the five phenotypes. To control for any potential population stratification, all analyses were stratified by race categories: Caucasian and African-American. Other racial categories were not considered because of the small numbers of those samples. We tested for Hardy-Weinberg equilibrium within both the Caucasian and African-American groups, and all subjects from a stratum were used in the analysis since all subjects had depression and the evaluated polymorphisms were not suspected to influence risk of depression.

We used unconditional logistic regression analysis to examine associations of the eleven genetic polymorphisms and each of the four phenotypic comparisons. These comparisons are (1) responder vs. non-responder, (2) remitter vs. non-responders, (3) specific responders vs. both non-responders and non-specific responders, and (4) specific responders vs. non-specific responders. Each polymorphism was modeled individually as gene-dosage effects in the regression models. This coding scheme was chosen because of its robustness to departure from the true additive genetic model (18). Regression analyses were performed either unadjusted or adjusted for potential confounding effects, including sex, age, education (years of school), months in current major depressive episode (MDE), and years since first MDE. We found that adjustment for potential confounders did not significantly influence the results, thus the values reported here are unadjusted. We estimated odds ratios (OR) and 95% confidence intervals (CIs) for the carriers of the minor allele versus non-carriers of the minor allele. Because of the large number of statistical tests, significance threshold was set at 0.01, and permutation tests were performed on any test that resulted in an asymptotic p value of 0.01 or less.

Association between haplotypes within the haplotype blocks and citalopram response were calculated using a score test implemented in the computer program HAPLO.SCORE (19). This test uses the expectation-maximization algorithm to estimate the posterior probability of each person's haplotype. These posterior probabilities are then used to calculate a person's expected haplotype score in the logistic regression analyses. All haplotypes with frequencies > 0.01 were simultaneously tested in the analysis. Global p values and individual haplotype p values were obtained. Statistical tests were performed in SAS version 8.2 or Splus version 6.2.1 statistical packages.

4.3 Results

4.3.1 Tagging SNP selection. We utilized the combined dataset of variant information from our previous resequencing (Chapter 3) and genotyping (Chapter 2) efforts to select maximally informative tagSNPs for use in our larger clinical population taking citalopram. The combined dataset consisted of 145 SNPs; 77 from resequencing, 52 from our previous genotyping effort, and 16 that were assayed using both methods. For tagSNP selection, we only used data from a subgroup of Caucasian individuals (N=75) in our patient population taking fluoxetine. Difficulties arise from attempting to predict rare genotypes (defined here as <10% minor allele frequency) or haplotypes (defined here as <1% population frequency) using a reduced tagging SNP set, as has been noted using other datasets and tagging methods (20;21). Attempts to tag rare SNPs resulted in the majority of these rare SNPs being selected as tagSNPs (Figure 4.1). The inclusion of rare SNPs almost doubled the number of tagging SNPs selected (28 for common SNPs vs. 51 for all SNPs). Similarly, for haplotype tagging methods such as the approach of Stram *et al.*, tagging rare recombinant haplotypes required large increases in tagging SNP selection. In several instances, rare haplotypes were not tagged accurately (i.e., R_h^2 <0.8) even when all SNPs within a block were selected as tagging SNPs (data not shown). Here, we thus limited our analysis of tagSNP performance to the tagging of common SNPs (N=71 SNPs) and common haplotypes.

In addition to serving as proxies for other SNPs, we sought to investigate how accurately these tagSNPs would infer the underlying haplotype structure. In order to aid haplotype tagging SNP selection we selected regions of limited haplotype diversity, also known as haplotype blocks. In total, eight haplotype blocks were identified, with an average length of 33 kb, using the chromosomal coverage criteria of Zhang *et al.* The *HTR2A* gene was composed of three blocks, while the *TPH2* gene had two blocks and the three other genes were all captured by a single haplotype block.

As shown in Figure 4.2, tagSNPs selected using Carlson et al.'s pairwise r^2 criteria predicted all the common haplotypes well in all blocks investigated (>0.75 average minimum R_h^2). The tagSNPs selected by the method of Stram et al. predicted all common haplotypes in all blocks accurately (>0.80 average minimum R_h^2), which is not surprising given that this method selects tagSNPs based solely on satisfying

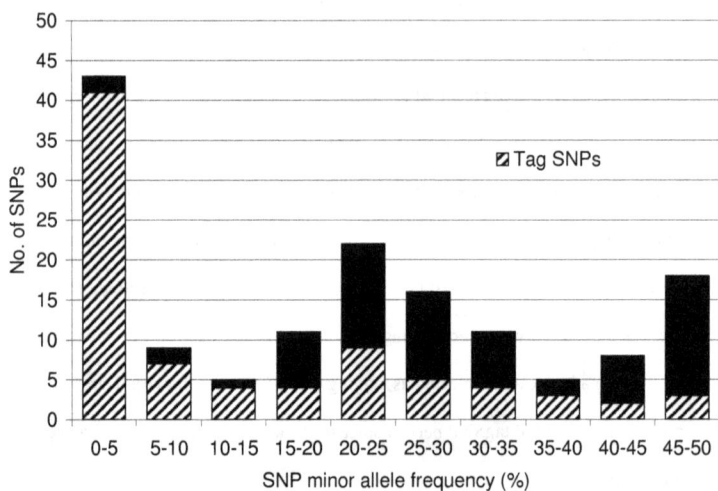

Figure 4.1. Effect of minor allele frequency on tagging SNP selection. The above histogram displays the number of SNPs (N=145 total) at each minor allele frequency bin (solid black bars). The striped bars indicate the number of SNPs, in each minor allele frequency bin, that were selected as tagSNPs using the method of Carlson *et al.* (6)

the R_h^2 threshold. In contrast, tagSNPs chosen using the pattern recognition approach of Ke *et al.* do not predict all common haplotypes well for 4 of the 8 blocks (<0.60 average minimum R_h^2). The three methods varied in their efficiency in reducing number of tagSNPs to be genotyped. The pattern recognition approach of Ke *et al.* was the most efficient, and selected 16 tagSNPs for the five genes out of a total of 71 common SNPs. The Stram *et al.* method selected 21 tagSNPs, and the Carlson *et al.* method selected 28 tagSNPs overall. Given that using a pairwise r^2 criteria is analytically straightforward and that the tagSNPs chosen will be sufficient in accurately reconstructing the underlying common haplotypes, we attempted to genotype the 28 tagSNPs selected by the method of Carlson et al in our clinical population taking citalopram (STAR*D). Of these 28 SNPs, a single SNP in the *HTR2A* gene (rs2246127) was out of Hardy-Weinberg equilibrium and thus dropped from the analysis.

4.3.2 Tagging SNP association to citalopram response. We sought to test two main hypotheses with the tagSNPs selected in these candidate genes using the response phenotypes described above. We first tested whether these variants were associated with overall response to citalopram by comparing responders to non-responders and remitters to non-responders. We also tested whether these variants affect "true" or specific drug response by comparing specific responders to non-responders and specific responders to non-specific responders. All analyses were stratified by self-reported ethnicity (Caucasian or African-American) to limit potential population stratification.

Table 4.3 shows the association results for our primary phenotypic comparison; response versus non-response. As can be seen, none of the tagSNPs were significantly associated with citalopram response at the p<0.01 threshold in

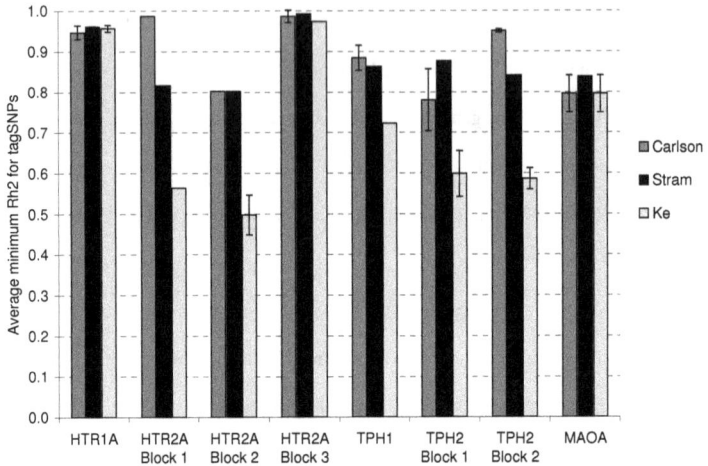

Figure 4.2. Accuracy of haplotype inference for three sets of tagging SNPs. Each of the eight haplotype blocks are shown on the x-axis. The minimum haplotype R_h^2 value for all common haplotypes reconstructed from each tagSNP set is shown on the y-axis. Due to the fact that methods of Carlson et al. (6) and Ke et al. (9) do not output a unique set of tagSNPs, average (± SD) minimum R_h^2 of all combinations of tagSNPs are shown.

this phenotypic comparison. The only variant to meet this threshold was an intronic SNP in the *HTR2A* gene (rs1923884) in a related phenotypic comparison; remitter versus non-responder (p<0.008, OR=0.72, 95% C.I. 0.55-0.93). This association was seen in the Caucasian subset, but was not significant within the African American samples (data not shown). No tagSNPs met our threshold for significance (p<0.01) in our "true" drug response comparisons; specific responders versus non-responders, and specific responders versus non-specific responders (Table 4.4).

As expected based on our tagSNP ascertainment, allelic association between the variants was low in our citalopram population, with no pairwise r^2 value greater than 0.8 in the STAR*D sample set. We inferred haplotypes within each haplotype block in the five candidate genes and tested them globally for association to citalopram response. No significant haplotypic associations were observed in any of the haplotype blocks using our four phenotypic comparisons (data not shown).

4.4 Discussion

In this chapter, we sought to test whether DNA variation in five serotonergic candidate genes is associated with clinical response to citalopram treatment. To accomplish this we used our previous genotype information and complete exon resequencing to select tagSNPs within these genes and then examined them in a large population taking citalopram. In our primary phenotypic, responders versus non-responders, no variants met our significance threshold (p<0.01). While a single SNP exceeded this threshold in a related phenotype comparison, remitters versus non-responders, the association is at best considered marginal given the large number of statistical tests that were performed. Additionally, no variants met our significance

		Responders (Resp, N=789) vs. non-responders (NR, N=501)				Remitters (Remit, N=669) vs. non-responders (NR=501)			
		MAF				MAF			
Gene	tagSNP	NR	Resp	p-value	Odds ratio (95% CI)	NR	Remit	p-value	Odds ratio (95% CI)
HTR1A	rs6295	0.48	0.47	-	-	0.48	0.47	-	-
HTR1A	rs1364043	0.22	0.21	-	-	0.22	0.22	-	-
HTR2A	rs731245	0.47	0.47	-	-	0.47	0.47	-	-
HTR2A	rs6313	0.42	0.40	-	-	0.42	0.39	-	-
HTR2A	rs2296973	0.30	0.32	-	-	0.30	0.31	-	-
HTR2A	rs927544	0.27	0.28	-	-	0.27	0.27	-	-
HTR2A	rs666693	0.19	0.20	-	-	0.19	0.20	-	-
HTR2A	rs2770296	0.25	0.29	0.07	1.13 (0.90, 1.43)	0.25	0.29	0.06	1.16 (0.91, 1.47)
HTR2A	rs1923884	0.15	0.12	0.02	0.75 (0.59, 0.97)	0.15	0.12	0.008	0.72 (0.55, 0.93)
HTR2A	rs1923882	0.25	0.23	-	-	0.25	0.23	-	-
HTR2A	rs6314	0.10	0.09	-	-	0.10	0.09	-	-
HTR2A	rs3125	0.16	0.14	-	-	0.16	0.14	-	-
TPH1	rs7130929	0.40	0.38	-	-	0.40	0.37	-	-
TPH1	rs623580	0.32	0.33	-	-	0.32	0.33	-	-
TPH1	rs684302	0.41	0.42	-	-	0.41	0.42	-	-
TPH1	rs211105	0.23	0.21	-	-	0.23	0.21	-	-
TPH1	rs211102	0.18	0.18	-	-	0.18	0.19	-	-
TPH1	rs2108977	0.45	0.44	-	-	0.45	0.44	-	-
TPH2	rs2129575	0.26	0.25	-	-	0.26	0.25	-	-
TPH2	rs2171363	0.43	0.42	-	-	0.43	0.42	-	-
TPH2	rs1007023	0.15	0.15	-	-	0.15	0.15	-	-
TPH2	rs1487278	0.21	0.22	-	-	0.21	0.23	-	-
TPH2	rs1487276	0.17	0.17	-	-	0.17	0.17	-	-
TPH2	rs1386487	0.40	0.36	0.08	0.87 (0.69, 1.10)	0.40	0.36	-	-
TPH2	rs17110747	0.15	0.15	-	-	0.15	0.15	-	-
TPH2	rs1872824	0.39	0.35	0.05	0.81 (0.64, 1.02)	0.39	0.36	-	-
MAOA	rs1465108	0.29	0.3	-	-	0.29	0.3	-	-

Table 4.3. Tagging SNP association results for the citalopram response and remission phenotype comparisons. Minor allele frequency in each phenotype group are shown, as well as the p-value and odds ratio for all SNPs with a p<0.1.

Gene	tagSNP	MAF		p-value	Odds ratio (95% CI)	MAF		p-value	Odds ratio (95% CI)
		NS	Spec			NS+NR	Spec		
HTR1A	rs6295	0.46	0.47	-	-	0.48	0.47	-	-
HTR1A	rs1364043	0.19	0.22	-	-	0.22	0.22	-	-
HTR2A	rs731245	0.43	0.47	-	-	0.46	0.47	-	-
HTR2A	rs6313	0.36	0.39	-	-	0.41	0.39	-	-
HTR2A	rs2296973	0.34	0.32	-	-	0.30	0.32	-	-
HTR2A	rs927544	0.30	0.28	-	-	0.28	0.28	-	-
HTR2A	rs666693	0.23	0.20	-	-	0.20	0.20	-	-
HTR2A	rs2770296	0.29	0.29	-	-	0.26	0.29	-	-
HTR2A	rs1923884	0.12	0.12	-	-	0.14	0.12	0.06	0.81 (0.62, 1.05)
HTR2A	rs1923882	0.23	0.23	-	-	0.24	0.23	-	-
HTR2A	rs6314	0.10	0.09	-	-	0.10	0.09	-	-
HTR2A	rs3125	0.13	0.14	-	-	0.16	0.14	-	-
TPH1	rs7130929	0.33	0.39	0.07	1.65 (1.13, 2.41)	0.39	0.39	-	-
TPH1	rs623580	0.33	0.34	-	-	0.33	0.34	-	-
TPH1	rs684302	0.45	0.40	-	-	0.42	0.40	-	-
TPH1	rs211105	0.18	0.22	-	-	0.22	0.22	-	-
TPH1	rs211102	0.19	0.18	-	-	0.18	0.18	-	-
TPH1	rs2108977	0.44	0.44	-	-	0.45	0.44	-	-
TPH2	rs2129575	0.27	0.25	-	-	0.26	0.25	-	-
TPH2	rs2171363	0.45	0.42	-	-	0.44	0.42	-	-
TPH2	rs1007023	0.15	0.15	-	-	0.15	0.15	-	-
TPH2	rs1487278	0.24	0.22	-	-	0.22	0.22	-	-
TPH2	rs1487276	0.17	0.18	-	-	0.17	0.18	-	-
TPH2	rs1386487	0.34	0.37	-	-	0.38	0.37	-	-
TPH2	rs17110747	0.16	0.15	-	-	0.16	0.15	-	-
TPH2	rs1872824	0.37	0.36	-	-	0.39	0.36	-	-
MAOA	rs1465108	0.34	0.27	0.05	0.66 (0.3, 0.95)	0.31	0.27	-	-

Table 4.4. Tagging SNP association results for the citalopram specific response phenotype comparisons. Minor allele frequency in each phenotype group are shown, as well as the p-value and odds ratio for all SNPs with a p<0.1.

threshold in our other phenotypic comparisons investigating association to "true", or specific drug response. Similar results were obtained using inferred haplotypes within these genes. Given that we had adequate power to detect reasonable effect sizes (Figure 4.3), it appears that variation in these five genes does not significantly influence patient response to citalopram.

We had previously reported an association to fluxoetine response for several of these variants, but none of them were significantly associated with citalopram response in our current study. Several factors could explain this difference, including different underlying mechanisms of action for the two drugs, differences in patient ascertainment between the two studies, cryptic population stratification, or simply Type I error. We attempted to control for population stratification in this study by analyzing the data within self-identified ethnic groups, as this has been shown to correlate well with marker allele frequencies (22).

One strength of this study is the comprehensive approach we took to selecting tagSNPs within these candidate genes using dense marker data in our small population taking fluoxetine. It could now be argued that simply using markers from the HapMap Project (24) would suffice, although there are several reasons why our approach had merit. First, the HapMap was not available when many of the experiments were carried out. Second, our resequencing provides finer granularity in our data, particularly for less common variants. Finally, the characteristics of the markers were measured in a population much like our test population, raising the possibility that the empirically tested marker set would be useful in the STAR*D dataset. Our coverage of variants within African American samples in this study was limited, due to the fact that our discovery sample was enriched with Caucasian samples. Our comparison of haplotype and SNP tagging methods revealed that the

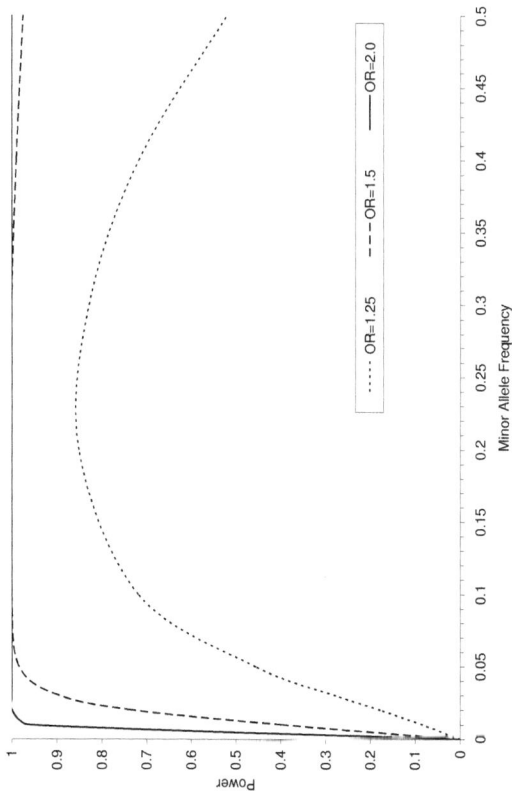

Figure 4.3. Power to detect association to categorical response to citalopram in the STAR*D population (N=1,914). On the y-axis is the power (1-β) of detecting an association at the various minor allele frequencies shown on the x-axis. Three different effect sizes (dominant ORs) are shown. Power was calculated using the method of Purcell et al (23). SNP's that were associated with response in the fluoxetine sample had ORs ranging from 2-5, thus we had adequate power to replicate these findings in the STARD population.

methods vary in the number of tagSNPs selected and their ability to accurately reconstruct common haplotypes. The pattern recognition approach to selecting haplotype tagging SNPs was the most efficient at reducing genotyping load, however within several blocks the tagSNPs could not accurately reconstruct the underlying haplotypes. This is not surprising given that this method does not take into account the uncertainty involved in predicting haplotypes from genotypic data. The R_h^2 method of Stram *et al.* accounts for this uncertainty, and selected a greater number of tagSNPs to be genotyped. The pairwise r^2 SNP tagging method of Carlson *et al.* was the least efficient at reducing genotyping costs. However, we were able to show that the tagSNPs selected using pairwise r^2 measures were sufficient to tag the common haplotypes as well. Given the computational simplicity of this method and since it allows us to test for both single locus and haplotypic effects, we chose to use the tagSNPs selected by this method in our citalopram population.

While we have attempted to capture the majority of common variation within these genes, current genotyping costs prohibit complete ascertainment of all variants. Interestingly, a recent study by McMahon *et al* which utilized the same STAR*D clinical population reported a significant association between a SNP in the *HTR2A* gene (rs7997012) and citalopram remission after interrogating 768 SNPs in 68 pharmacodynamic candidate genes (25). This intronic SNP was not initially included in our study, though we subsequently genotyped it in our STAR*D sample. This SNP was not in significant LD with any of our tagSNPs within this gene (max $r^2 = 0.19$). In fact, Phase 2 HapMap data shows that only one variant (rs9567732) within 1Mb of this SNP has moderate ($r^2 > 0.80$) LD with it. Analysis of this SNP using our phenotypic definitions and statistical methods also showed modest association with citalopram remission (p<0.002), however, our level of significance was two orders of magnitude less than reported by the McMahon group (p<0.00004). This is largely due to the fact that we stratified our analyses by race, whereas their primary analysis is performed on the entire sample. We stratified our analysis since both remission rate and the minor allele frequency of rs7997012 are strongly correlated with self-reported race in the STAR*D sample. Thus, confounding due to population stratification seems to increase the significance of their finding, though within racial subgroups, the variant is still nominally associated with remission. As always, replication of this finding in an independent sample is critical, and because the effect size of the variant was small, additional risk variants are required in order to utilize genetic information in clinical decision making.

In summary, our study has attempted to broadly investigate these five serotonin genes for association to citalopram response in a large patient population. Using both single locus and haplotype tests, none of the polymorphisms we interrogated appear to be strongly associated with citalopram response or response specificity in the STAR*D population. Given that little is known about exactly how SSRIs exert their antidepressant effects *in vivo*, interrogation of DNA variation in other neuronal pathways or across the entire genome may be required to gain further insight.

4.5 References

1.   Trivedi MH, Rush AJ, Wisniewski SR, Nierenberg AA, Warden D, Ritz L, Norquist G, Howland RH, Lebowitz B, McGrath PJ, Shores-Wilson K, Biggs MM, Balasubramani GK, Fava M, Team DS. Evaluation of outcomes with citalopram for depression using measurement-based care in STAR*D: Implications for clinical practice. *Am J Psychiatry* 2006; 163(1):28-40.

2.   Rush AJ, Trivedi MH, Wisniewski SR, Stewart JW, Nierenberg AA, Thase ME, Ritz L, Biggs MM, Warden D, Luther JF, Shores-Wilson K, Niederehe G, Fava M, the STAR. Bupropion-SR, Sertraline, or Venlafaxine-XR after failure of SSRIs for depression. *N Engl J Med* 2006; 354(12):1231-1242.

3.   Rush AJ, Trivedi MH, Wisniewski SR, Nierenberg AA, Stewart JW, Warden D, Niederehe G, Thase ME, Lavori PW, Lebowitz BD, McGrath PJ, Rosenbaum JF, Sackeim HA, Kupfer DJ, Luther J, Fava M. Acute and longer-term outcomes in depressed outpatients requiring one or several treatment steps: a STAR*D report. *Am J Psychiatry* 2006; 163(11):1905-1917.

4.   Peters EJ, Slager SL, McGrath PJ, Knowles JA, Hamilton SP. Investigation of serotonin-related genes in antidepressant response. *Mol Psychiatry* 2004; 9(9):879-889.

5.   Kraft JB, Peters EJ, Slager SL, Jenkins GD, Reinalda MS, McGrath PJ, Hamilton SP. Analysis of association between the serotonin transporter and antidepressant response in a large clinical sample. *Biol Psychiatry* 2006; advanced online publication.

6.   Carlson CS, Eberle MA, Rieder MJ, Yi Q, Kruglyak L, Nickerson DA. Selecting a maximally informative set of single-nucleotide polymorphisms for association analyses using linkage disequilibrium. *Am J Hum Genet* 2004; 74(1):106-120.

7.   Sebastiani P, Lazarus R, Weiss ST, Kunkel LM, Kohane IS, Ramoni MF. Minimal haplotype tagging. *PNAS* 2003; 100(17):9900-9905.

8.   Stram DO, Haiman CA, Hirschhorn JN, Altshuler D, Kolonel LN, Henderson BE, Pike MC. Choosing haplotype-tagging SNPS based on unphased genotype data using a preliminary sample of unrelated subjects with an example from the Multiethnic Cohort Study. *Hum Hered* 2003; 55(1):27-36.

9.   Ke X, Cardon LR. Efficient selective screening of haplotype tag SNPs. *Bioinformatics* 2003; 19(2):287-288.

10.   Fava M, Rush AJ, Trivedi MH, Nierenberg AA, Thase ME, Sackeim HA, Quitkin FM, Wisniewski S, Lavori PW, Rosenbaum JF, Kupfer DJ. Background and rationale for the sequenced treatment alternatives to relieve depression (STAR*D) study. *Psychiatr Clin North Am* 2003; 26(2):457-94, x.

11.   Rush AJ, Fava M, Wisniewski SR, Lavori PW, Trivedi MH, Sackeim HA, Thase ME, Nierenberg AA, Quitkin FM, Kashner TM. Sequenced treatment alternatives to relieve depression (STAR*D): rationale and design. *Controlled Clinical Trials* 2004; 25(1):119-142.

12.   Rush AJ, Trivedi MH, Ibrahim HM, Carmody TJ, Arnow B, Klein DN, Markowitz JC, Ninan PT, Kornstein S, Manber R. The 16-Item quick inventory of depressive symptomatology (QIDS), clinician rating (QIDS-C), and self-report (QIDS-SR): a psychometric evaluation in patients with chronic major depression. *Biol Psychiatry* 2003; 54(5):573-583.

13.   Ross DC, Quitkin FM, Klein DF. A typological model for estimation of drug and placebo effects in depression. *J Clin Psychopharmacol* 2002; 22(4):414-418.

14.   Quitkin FM, Rabkin JD, Markowitz JM, Stewart JW, McGrath, PJ, Harrison W. Use of pattern analysis to identify true drug response. A replication. *Arch Gen Psychiatry* 1987; 44(3):259-264.

15.   Stewart JW, Quitkin FM, McGrath PJ, Amsterdam J, Fava M, Fawcett J, Reimherr F, Rosenbaum J, Beasley C, Roback P. Use of pattern analysis to predict differential relapse of remitted patients with major depression during 1 year of treatment with fluoxetine or placebo. *Arch Gen Psychiatry* 1998; 55(4):334-343.

16.   Carlson CS, Eberle MA, Rieder MJ, Yi Q, Kruglyak L, Nickerson DA. Selecting a maximally informative set of single-nucleotide polymorphisms for association analyses using linkage disequilibrium. *Am J Hum Genet* 2004; 74(1):106-120.

17.   Zhang K, Jin L. HaploBlockFinder: haplotype block analyses. *Bioinformatics* 2003; 19(10):1300-1301.

18.   Freidlin B, Zheng G, Li Z, Gastwirth JL. Trend tests for case-control studies of genetic markers: power, sample size and robustness. *Hum Hered* 2002; 53(3):146-152.

19.   Schaid DJ, Rowland CM, Tines DE, Jacobson RM, Poland GA. Score tests for association between traits and haplotypes when linkage phase is ambiguous. *Am J Hum Genet* 2002; 70(2):425-434.

20.   Weale ME, Depondt C, Macdonald SJ, Smith A, Lai PS, Shorvon SD, Wood NW, Goldstein DB. Selection and evaluation of tagging SNPs in the neuronal-sodium-channel gene SCN1A: implications for linkage-disequilibrium gene mapping. *Am J Hum Genet* 2003; 73(3):551-565.

21.   Goldstein DB, Ahmadi KR, Weale ME, Wood NW. Genome scans and candidate gene approaches in the study of common diseases and variable drug responses. *Trends Genet* 2003; 19(11):615-622.

22.   Tang H, Quertermous T, Rodriguez B, Kardia SL, Zhu X, Brown A, Pankow JS, Province MA, Hunt SC, Boerwinkle E, Schork NJ, Risch NJ. Genetic structure, self-identified race/ethnicity, and confounding in case-control association studies. *Am J Hum Genet* 2005; 76(2):268-275.

23.   Purcell S, Cherny SS, Sham PC. Genetic Power Calculator: design of linkage and association genetic mapping studies of complex traits. *Bioinformatics* 2003; 19(1):149-150.

24.   The International HapMap Consortium. A haplotype map of the human genome. *Nature* 2005; 437(7063):1299-1320.

25.   McMahon FJ, Buervenich S, Charney D, Lipsky R, Rush AJ, Wilson AF, Sorant AJ, Papanicolaou GJ, Laje G, Fava M, Trivedi MH, Wisniewski SR, Manji H. Variation in the gene encoding the serotonin 2A receptor is associated with outcome of antidepressant treatment. *Am J Hum Genet* 2006; 78(5):804-814.

CHAPTER 5

TESTING FUNCTIONAL VARIATION IN PHARMACOKINETIC GENES FOR

ASSOCIATION TO CITALOPRAM RESPONSE AND TOLERANCE[*]

5.1 Introduction

Significant inter-individual variation exists in clinical response to and

tolerance of antidepressant medication. Common genetic variation may be partly

responsible for these phenotypic differences. The use of genotype information in

clinical psychopharmacology could potentially help clinicians avoid the standard trial

and error approach, and allow a more efficient way to maximize efficacy and

minimize toxicity (1) as is done in certain situations with cancer treatment (2).

Drug metabolism and transport genes such as *CYP2D6* and *CYP2C19* are

obvious pharmacogenetic candidate genes given their known interaction with drugs

like selective serotonin reuptake inhibitors (SSRI) and their metabolites *in vivo* (3).

For example, Yin *et al.* found that homozygous carriers of the non-functional allele of

CYP2C19 show a 42% decrease in clearance of the SSRI citalopram compared to that

of homozygous carriers of the wild type allele (4). Moreover, several of these

pharmacokinetic genes harbor common variants that have been shown to impair

enzyme function (5).

Despite these known *in vivo* relationship between antidepressant medications

and pharmacogenetic genes, few epidemiological studies investigating the

relationship between antidepressant response and pharmacokinetic gene variants have

been carried out. In a prospective study of subjects taking the SSRI paroxetine,

CYP2D6 genotype was not associated with side effect burden (6). Another recent

---

[*] This work has been submitted for publication (Peters E.J., Slager S.L., Kraft J.B., Jenkins G.D., Reinalda M.S., McGrath P.J., Hamilton S.P. 2007 "Pharmacokinetic genes do not influence response or tolerance to citalopram in the STAR*D sample.")

147

study found that *CYP2D6* genotype does not influence the frequency of gastrointestinal side effects, although when *CYP2D6* genotype is combined with a serotonin 2A receptor polymorphism, the authors did observe such an association (7). Despite the equivocal results of these studies, some investigators have advocated the use of pharmacokinetic enzyme variant information to guide clinical therapy of SSRI, particularly by adjustment of the dose prescribed (8;9). Here, we investigate the potential role of five pharmacokinetic genes on the response to and tolerance of citalopram using a large clinical sample of depressed patients who are enrolled in the Sequenced Treatment Alternatives to Relieve Depression (STAR*D) study (10).

The majority of the metabolism of citalopram occurs through two sequential N-methylations, the first to form desmethylcitalopram (DCT) and the second to form didesmethylcitalopram (DDCT) (11). The first step is primarily catalyzed by the CYP2C19 enzyme with some contribution from CYP3A4, and the second step is primarily catalyzed by the CYP2D6 enzyme (12). P-glycoprotein (encoded by *ABCB1*) is thought to contribute to the control of citalopram flux across the blood brain barrier (13). At steady state, DCT and DDCT are half and one-tenth as abundant, respectively, in plasma compared to unchanged citalopram (11). Furthermore, DCT and DDCT are 0.12 fold and 0.08 fold less potent, respectively, at inhibiting the serotonin transport *in vitro* than the parent compound (14) (Figure 5.1). The combination of low plasma concentrations and weak inhibition of the serotonin transporter suggest that DCT and DDCT do not contribute significantly to citalopram's antidepressant effects.

5.2 Methods

5.2.1 STAR*D clinical sample. Subjects are those enrolled in STAR*D who consented to give DNA (N=1,953). The STAR*D trial was a large NIMH-sponsored

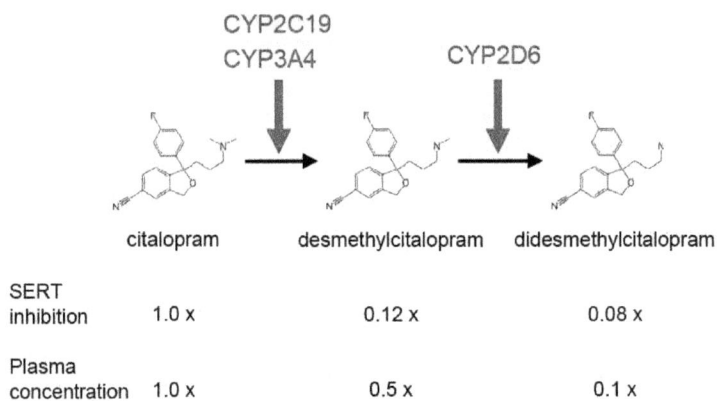

Figure 5.1. Metabolism of citalopram by CYP enzymes. Steady state plasma levels and *in vitro* serotonin transporter (SERT) inhibition are shown relative to the parent compound.

treatment trial involving 4,041 subjects that was designed to assess effectiveness of antidepressant treatments in generalizable samples, and to determine outcomes for outpatients with non-psychotic major depressive disorder (MDD) treated with citalopram. The study design and methods for this clinical trial are reviewed in Chapter 4 as well as in the literature (15). Further demographic information on the cohort that consented to give DNA is presented in our previous work (16) (Table 4.1). The aim of STAR*D was to prospectively determine which of a number of treatments are beneficial for subjects experiencing an unsatisfactory response to citalopram. To increase the generalizability of the findings, STAR*D utilized broad inclusion criteria and enrolled an ethnically diverse population (10). Diagnosis was made using the Psychiatric Diagnostic Screening Questionnaire, and depressive symptoms were assessed with the 16-item Quick Inventory of Depressive Symptomatology (Self-Report [QIDS-SR] version) (17) collected at clinic visits. Subjects meeting criteria and providing consent were administered citalopram for 12 weeks of treatment with vigorous dosing (20-60mg/day). The subset of subjects who provided DNA samples was 61.8% female, and was 78.1% Caucasian, 16.1% African-American, and 5.8% other races (16). Hispanics accounted for 14.0% of the sample. The average citalopram dose at study exit was 45.5 mg (s.d. = 15.7). Subjects were consented for genetic studies as part of the National Institute of Mental Health's Human Genetic Initiative, and the work described here was approved by the institutional review board of the University of California, San Francisco.

5.2.2 Phenotypic definitions. We defined six phenotypes to evaluate citalopram response and tolerability. The first two were **responders** and **non-responders**: responders are subjects who had at least 42 days of treatment and whose QIDS-SR score on their final clinical visit shows ≥50% reduction in score; the remaining subjects, who also had at least 42 days of treatment, were then considered non-responders. The $\geq 50\%$ reduction in symptom severity on the $HRSD_{17}$ is the conventional definition of response in clinical trials. We used the QIDS-SR score to estimate severity since all subjects had this rating and it correlates highly with the 17-item Hamilton Rating Scale for Depression ($HRSD_{17}$) score (17). We required this 42 day threshold to ensure an adequate exposure to citalopram and to enhance the power to find associations between genotype and response by reducing potential heterogeneity. The third phenotype was **remission**, defined as a final QIDS-SR score ≤ 5. Our **specific** response phenotype is based on our attempt to further reduce heterogeneity by attempting to separate placebo response from true drug response in antidepressant trials (18). Some response to antidepressant medication is a placebo response, which we posit may have either no genetic determinant or a different genetic underpinning than "true" drug response. Thus it is of interest to limit our definition of response to true pharmacologic response rather than placebo response. For these phenotypes, a "specific" pattern of response was defined by persistence, or the maintenance of response for the remainder of the study once it was attained. Previous studies considered "specific" patterns to be further characterized by delayed response, i.e., after the first two weeks (19). We were unable to employ this criterion because the STAR*D study design did not include ratings before week two. We defined persistent, or **"specific"** responders, as those subjects who had a sustained response at all consecutive visits following the first visit with response, as measured by $\geq 50\%$ reduction in QIDS-SR scores. Those whose response occurred only at the last visit were removed from the analysis. Note that "specific" responders are a subset of responders (as defined by the response phenotype above). Moreover, because visits were at least two weeks apart, we assumed that intervening weeks were characterized by the response defined by the previous visit. Our tolerance outcome was based on study exit data; all patients who continued with citalopram at the end of STAR*D Level 1 treatment were considered **tolerant**, while patients who refused to continue citalopram or left the study due to side effects were considered **intolerant**. For those who left Level 1 for further treatment but did not want to continue with citalopram, their phenotype was probably tolerant, probably intolerant, or intolerant based on the level of side effects at the study exit based on the Global Rating of Side Effect Burden (20). In order to reduce heterogeneity, we did not use subjects who were considered probably tolerant or probably intolerant.

5.2.3 Molecular methods. Several cytochrome P450 genes (*CYP2C19*, *CYP2D6*, *CYP3A4*, *CYP3A5*) as well as the P-glycoprotein transporter protein (*ABCB1*) are thought to be involved in the metabolism and distribution of citalopram, based on human and animal model pharmacokinetic studies (12;13). We chose to examine DNA variants in cytochrome P450 genes that cause or are suspected to cause severe functional changes in the targeted proteins. We also investigated three common SNPs in the ABCB1 gene (C1236T, G2677T, and C3435T) that have been associated with treatment outcome in acute myeloid leukemia patients and reduced P-glycoprotein expression *in vivo*, though results are not unequivocal (21;22).

Patients were genotyped for *CYP3A5*3C, all three *CYP2C19* variants (*2, *3, *17), and all three *ABCB1* variants using commercially available 5' exonuclease fluorescence (Taqman) assays (see section 4.2.7 for laboratory assay conditions). *CYP2D6*5 deletion status was determined using a previously published tetra-primer long range PCR assay (23). All other *CYP2D6* alleles (*3, *4, *6, *7, *8, *9) were determined by first specifically amplifying the *CYP2D6* gene as a 5.1kb long range PCR product (as described in (23)) followed by direct sequencing of two regions

Gene	Variant	Caucasian	African-American	Enzyme function in vivo
CYP2D6	*3	0.02	0.003	none
CYP2D6	*4	0.19	0.07	none
CYP2D6	*5	0.03	0.06	none
CYP2D6	*6	0.01	0.003	none
CYP2D6	*7	0.0003	0.002	none
CYP2D6	*8	-	-	none
CYP2D6	*9	0.03	0.005	decreased
CYP3A4	*1B	0.04	0.65	unknown
CYP3A5	*3C	0.09	0.70	decreased
CYP2C19	*2	0.13	0.19	none
CYP2C19	*3	-	0.02	none
CYP2C19	*17	0.21	0.20	increased
ABCB1	C1236T	0.44	0.19	unknown
ABCB1	G2677T	0.44	0.08	unknown
ABCB1	C3435T	0.51	0.21	unknown
CYP2D6	PM	0.05	0.02	none
CYP2C19	PM	0.02	0.02	none

Table 5.1. List of genotyped variants in pharmacokinetic genes. Variants are listed by gene, accepted nomenclature (http://www.cypalleles.ki.se/ for cytochrome P450 genes), allele frequencies in the STAR*D sample, and known functional status of the variant. PM, poor metabolizer, defined as described in Methods.

containing exons 3-4 (sequencing primer: AAAGAGTGGGCCCTGTGACCAGCT)

and exons 5-6 (sequencing primer: GGGTGTCCCAGCAAAGTTCATGG). This two

step amplification procedure was preformed in order to avoid non-specific

amplification of the *CYP2D6* pseudogene located near the *CYP2D6* gene.

CYP3A4*1B genotype was determined by direct sequencing of a 320bp PCR product

that specifically amplifies the 5' proximal region of the *CYP3A4* gene (24). A

synopsis of the 15 variants is shown in Table 5.1. Direct sequencing genotypes were

scored using Mutation Surveyor v2.61.

5.2.4 Statistical methods. To reduce Type I error, we relied on a two-stage design

for analysis (25). Within each ethnic group, gender, and response to citalopram

(using only our responder and nonresponder phenotypes), we randomly split our

subjects *a priori* into a discovery set and validation set. Within each set, we stratified

all analyses by self-reported ethnicity due to the large allele frequency differences and

phenotype prevalence differences between ethnic groups. Only the two largest ethnic

groups (Caucasian and African-American) were analyzed. Hardy-Weinberg

equilibrium was evaluated for each SNP within the discovery set using all participants

within each ethnic group. This is because all subjects had depression, and we do not

suspect the variants to influence risk of depression. No SNPs were found to violate

Hardy-Weinberg equilibrium using a Bonferroni-corrected threshold. We used

unconditional logistic regression analysis to examine associations between each

genetic polymorphisms and each phenotypic comparison. Comparisons performed

were: 1) *responders* vs. *non-responders*, 2) *remitters* vs. *non-responders*, 3) *specific

responders* vs. *non-responders*, and 4) *tolerant* vs. *intolerant*. Table 5.2 displays the

sample sizes of our phenotypic comparisons and race and gender information for each

group. Each polymorphism was modeled individually as gene-dosage effects in the regression models, and odds ratios (OR) and 95% confidence intervals were estimated. For the CYP2D6 and CYP2C19 genes, we also modeled the putative metabolism status of the subjects as follows. Individuals with two (phase known) non-functional alleles in these genes were considered poor metabolizers (PMs), all other genotypes were considered extensive metabolizers (EMs). Ultra rapid metabolizers (UMs) were not detectable by our genotyping methodology. Association between haplotypes and the phenotypes were calculated using a score test implemented in the computer program HAPLO.SCORE (26). Pair-wise interactions among all independent SNPs were tested using logistic regression. A likelihood ratio test was used to test for significance of the interaction effect. Only those SNPs with a p-value of <0.05 from the single SNP analyses in the discovery set were evaluated in the validation set. Those SNPs in the validation set that had a p-value <0.05 and the same directionality of association as that in the screening set were reported as statistically significant. We used survival analysis to examine whether metabolizer status influenced the ability to complete the trial. Survival curves were generated by the method of Kaplan-Meier, and differences between PM and EM curves were tested using the log rank statistic. We also examined the relationship between metabolizer status and citalopram dose, comparing final dose between extensive and poor metabolizers at the CYP2D6 and CYP2C19 loci with a t-test.

5.3 Results

Patients were genotyped for 15 polymorphisms in the *CYP2D6*, *CYP2C19*, *CYP3A4*, *CYP3A5*, and *ABCB1* genes. We compared genotype frequencies between responders and non-responders, remitters and non-responders, and specific responders and non-responders within each racial subgroup. Note that remitters and specific responders

155

Variable	Discovery Set								Validation Set							
	Pheno 1[a]		Pheno 2[b]		Pheno 3[c]		Pheno 4[d]		Pheno 1[a]		Pheno 2[b]		Pheno 3[c]		Pheno 4[d]	
	Yes N(%)	No N(%)	Yes N(%)	No N(%)	Yes N(%)	No N(%)	Yes N(%)	No N(%)	Yes N(%)	No N(%)	Yes N(%)	No N(%)	Yes N(%)	No N(%)	Yes N(%)	No N(%)
Ethnicity																
African Amer.	66 (51.2)	63 (48.8)	52 (45.2)	63 (54.8)	40 (38.8)	63 (61.2)	89 (90.8)	9 (9.2)	64 (52.5)	58 (47.5)	48 (45.3)	58 (54.7)	37 (39.0)	58 (61.0)	86 (86.9)	13 (13.1)
Caucasian	395 (60.6)	257 (39.4)	331 (56.3)	257 (43.7)	287 (52.8)	257 (47.2)	514 (91.0)	51 (9.0)	404 (61.4)	254 (38.6)	348 (57.8)	254 (42.2)	272 (51.7)	254 (48.3)	554 (81.6)	125 (18.4)
Gender																
Female	288 (59.8)	194 (40.2)	239 (55.2)	194 (44.8)	202 (51.0)	194 (49.0)	382 (93.9)	25 (6.1)	297 (61.6)	185 (38.4)	253 (57.8)	185 (42.2)	199 (51.8)	185 (48.2)	400 (83.5)	79 (16.5)
Male	173 (57.9)	126 (42.1)	144 (53.3)	126 (46.7)	125 (49.8)	126 (50.2)	221 (86.3)	35 (13.7)	171 (57.4)	127 (42.6)	143 (53.0)	127 (47.0)	110 (46.4)	127 (53.6)	240 (80.3)	59 (19.7)

a. Responder vs. Non-responder
b. Remitter vs. Non-responder
c. Specific responder vs. Non-responder
d. Tolerant vs. Intolerant

Table 5.2. Sample sizes and frequency distribution of race and gender in the discovery and validation sets for each phenotype comparison.

are subsets of responders. We also compared genotype frequencies of subjects

intolerant to citalopram to those who could tolerant the medication. Table 5.2

displays the frequency distribution of the phenotypes by ethnicity among subjects for

the discovery and validation sets. Because one of our criteria for splitting our sample

was based on the response/non-response phenotypes, the distribution of response and

non-response are similar between the discovery and validation set. In the discovery

set, we found seven variants to be associated ($p < 0.05$) with citalopram response or

tolerance. All but one of these were found in the African-American ethnic group.

However, none of these SNPs were replicated in our validation set (Table 5.3). It is

of note that the point estimates for the odds ratios for nearly all of these variants

switched directionality in the second stage, most likely as a result of small samples

sizes and the low allele frequencies of those variants. Similar non-significant results

were obtained using haplotype testing (results not shown). CYP2D6 or CYP2C19

metabolizer status (PM vs. EM) was also not associated with citalopram response or

tolerance in the first stage (results not shown). We also found no evidence for

interaction ($P > 0.05$) between the variants in any of the genes tested (results not

shown). We further sought to determine if metabolizer genotype was correlated with

other clinical variables of interest, namely the dosage of citalopram and the length of

time a subject would continue with citalopram treatment. For all subjects, regardless

of outcome or length of trial, dose was not correlated with CYP2D6 or CYP2C19

metabolizer status (Table 5.4). Additionally, CYP2C19 or CYP2D6 metabolizer

status did not significantly influence the subject's ability to remain in the trial (Figure

5.2).

5.4 Discussion

157

There is growing interest in the utility of pharmacokinetic gene polymorphism screening in psychopharmacological treatment, particularly with antipsychotic medications and older antidepressant agents (5). Others have further argued that the use of most psychotropics could be impacted by DNA variants in pharmacokinetic genes, with decisions about which drug to use, as well as the appropriate dosing, based on genotypic information (8;9). The pharmacokinetics of many SSRIs, including citalopram, are affected by *CYP2D6* and *CYP2C19* genotype status, although there is no evidence regarding how plasma levels of citalopram influence clinical efficacy (27). For example, CYP2C19 poor metabolizers show a 42% decrease in citalopram clearance when compared to homozygous extensive metabolizers, yet there was no difference in side effects Despite the intuitive appeal of ascribing differences in drug tolerance and efficacy to variation in pharmacokinetic genes (9;28), no adequately powered studies have been published that consistently report a significant clinical effect. Considerable debate exists regarding the relevance of drug metabolizing enzymes for the clinical pharmacology of SSRIs (11). The flat dose-response curve and wide toxicity index argue against a strong relationship between plasma levels and clinical response (29). This appears to be the case for citalopram, which has few drug-drug interactions based on in vitro and in vivo studies (12). Nevertheless, polymorphisms in enzymes involved in citalopram metabolism, such as CYP2C19 and CYP2D6, do alter citalopram disposition (4;30-32). For example, in one study of seven non-responders to citalopram, six of seven were extensive metabolizers for CYP2D6 and all seven were CYP2C19 extensive metabolizers (33). When given an inhibitor of these two enzymes, citalopram serum levels rose in all seven subjects, with six of them showing substantial clinical improvement. These data suggest that enzymes involved in citalopram metabolism

Ethnicity	Phenotypic comparison	Gene	Variant	Discovery set p-value (OR, 95% CI)	Validation set p-value (OR, 95% CI)
Caucasian	Tolerant vs. intolerant	CYP2C19	*2	0.005 (0.44, 0.24 - 0.81)	0.86 (1.00, 0.63 - 1.57)
African Amer.	Responders vs. non-responders	ABCB1	C3435T	0.01 (0.36, 0.17 - 0.75)	0.59 (1.51, 0.70 - 3.26)
African Amer.	Remitters vs. non-responders	ABCB1	C3435T	0.02 (0.36, 0.16 - 0.78)	0.85 (1.28, 0.56 - 2.93)
African Amer.	Specific responders vs. non-responders	CYP2D6	*5	0.03 (4.44, 1.07 - 18.39)	0.32 (0.45, 0.09 - 2.37)
African Amer.	Specific responders vs. non-responders	CYP2D6	*4	0.04 (0.26, 0.05 - 1.23)	0.96 (1.24, 0.35 - 4.41)
African Amer.	Specific responders vs. non-responders	ABCB1	C3435T	0.02 (0.40, 0.17 - 0.93)	0.71 (1.39, 0.58 - 3.35)
African Amer.	Tolerant vs. intolerant	CYP3A5	*3	0.04 (0.32, 0.08 - 1.37)	0.33 (1.57, 0.48 - 5.07)

Table 5.3. Single locus results for tests that were significant (p<0.05) in the discovery sample set. Significance was assessed using logistic regression, and odds ratios (OR) and confidence intervals (CI) shown are for minor allele carrier versus non-carrier. No variants were significantly associated in both the discovery and validation sets.

Table 5.4 a)

Metabolizer status	Mean final dose (s.d.)	p-value
CYP2C19 EM	45.3 (15.7)	0.13
CYP2C19 PM	40.7 (16.4)	
CYP2D6 EM	45.4 (15.8)	0.25
CYP2D6 PM	43.2 (16.8)	

Table 5.4 b)

Metabolizer status	Mean final dose (s.d.)	p-value
CYP2C19 EM	46.7 (15.6)	0.87
CYP2C19 PM	45.7 (15.1)	
CYP2D6 EM	46.7 (15.7)	0.30
CYP2D6 PM	53.3 (10.3)	

Table 5.4. Effect of metabolizer status on final citalopram dose prescribed. Mean final dose (mg) for each metabolizer group is shown, along with the standard deviation (s.d.) and significance level assessed using student's t-test. Results are shown for the Caucasian subgroup (a), as well as the African-American subset (b).

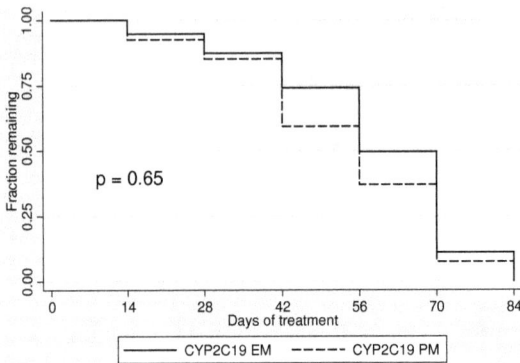

Figure 5.2 a)

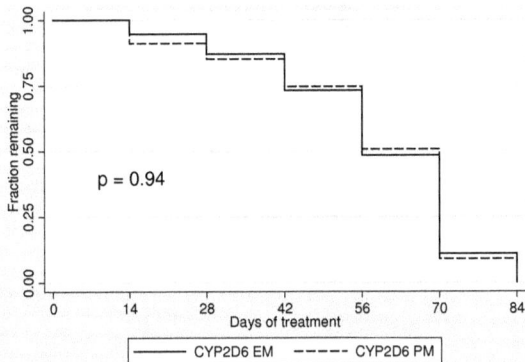

Figure 5.2 b)

Figure 5.2. Survival curves displaying fraction of subjects remaining in the trial, separated by cytochrome P450 metabolizer status. a) Subjects who were poor metabolizers (PM) for CYP2C19 were not significantly more likely to drop out of the trial earlier than extensive metabolizers (EM). b) Similar non-significant results were observed for subjects who were CYP2D6 PMs. Results displayed are for the Caucasian subgroup, similar results were obtained using the African American subgroup.

may contribute to response, at least in some extensive metabolizers. There are no similar data regarding side effects, although a sizable (n=749) Swedish study found no difference in citalopram or desmethylcitalopram levels between those experiencing a number of common side effects compared and those who did not (34).

The size of the STAR*D study provides a clinical sample with statistical power to detect moderately sized genetic influences. In this study, we detected no significant association between any of the polymorphisms and our treatment phenotypes. Our two-stage analysis allowed us to control Type I error by requiring validation of our results in a second sample. However, by splitting our sample as such, we sacrificed statistical power. For our response phenotype in the discovery set, we had 80% power to detect a minimum detectable odds ratio of 1.9 assuming an allele frequency of 0.05 and 5% significance level and using our Caucasian sample. The minimum detectable odds ratio increased to 2.74 for the tolerant phenotype. Given the lack of a dose-response relationship with citalopram in the literature, we expected that the results for the response phenotypes would not be significant. The negative association results for the tolerance phenotype in our Caucasian sample, however, were unexpected, as alterations of circulating drug or metabolite levels could conceivably lead to medication side effects and intolerance (27), although the power to detect small effects with this phenotype was limited. It is possible that genetic influence on a patient's medication tolerance is derived largely from pharmacodynamic as opposed to pharmacokinetic gene variation, as observed in study of paroxetine tolerance by Murphy *et al* (6).

The study described here has several limitations. Given the heterogenous sample, population stratification may be a potential explanation for our negative findings, with true associations being obscured by unobserved population sub-

162

structure. However, population studies have found that self-reported ethnicity is a close surrogate for underlying genetic ancestry information (35). We limited our genotyping of pharmacokinetic candidate genes to known, deleterious alleles that are common in Caucasian populations. In order to comprehensively screen these genes, rare and functionally unknown variants would need to be genotyped. The STAR*D clinical study, while large and broad in scope, was not designed for pharmacogenetic studies of this type. For instance, citalopram was chosen partly due to its lower potential for influence by pharmacokinetic polymorphism. Citalopram dosage was also not fixed, though the majority of subjects (78%) were receiving 40-60mg per day at the end of the study. The final citalopram dosage prescribed was not influenced by the subject's genotype status. This is consistent with work carried out with many of the same functional DNA variants in the Clinical Antipsychotic Trials of Intervention Effectiveness (CATIE) study, in which there was no association to dosing, efficacy, or tolerability to five antipsychotics (Iris Grossman and David Goldstein, personal communication). This observation is particularly interesting in that others have noted a strong correlation between maximum prescribed dose of phenytoin or carbemazepine in epilepsy and genetic variants in *CYP2C9* or *SCN1A* , suggesting the utility of clinical adjustment of dose in response to genotype (36). An additional limitation involves the allowance of concomitant medications in the STAR*D trial that potentially interfere with or accelerate the metabolism of citalopram. Without having data on co-administered medications, we were unable to control for this theoretical drug-drug interaction effect. It is noteworthy that the analysis of the CATIE study indicates that using concomitant medications known to alter metabolic status did not alter the results. Additionally, circulating concentrations of citalopram or citalopram metabolites were not obtained, which might have been useful as a proxy measure of compliance. Finally, our findings regarding citalopram may not be generalizable to other SSRI's, each of which has a unique metabolic disposition. Any broadly administered pharmacogenetic test will have to tolerate similar limitations in order to be clinically useful. Thus, at least for citalopram, it appears to be premature to advocate routine pharmacokinetic gene analysis for dose adjustment or clinical decision making.

In summary, here we have tested known functional variation in relevant pharmacokinetic gene for association to citalopram response and tolerance. Using a two stage study design and the STAR*D clinical population, none of these variants were significantly associated with clinical outcome in both our discovery and validation sample sets. Furthermore, combinations of these variants in the form of predicted metabolizer status for CYP2D6 and CYP2C19 (EM vs. PM) were not associated with clinical outcome. Final prescribed citalopram dose and length of time in trial was also not associated with pharmacokinetic gene variants. Thus, this study does not support a strong role for common pharmacokinetic gene variants in patient outcome from treatment with citalopram.

5.5 References

1.   Goldstein DB. Pharmacogenetics in the laboratory and the clinic. *N Engl J Med* 2003; 348(6):553-556.

2.   Eichelbaum M, Ingelman-Sundberg M, Evans WE. Pharmacogenomics and individualized drug therapy. *Annual Review of Medicine* 2006; 57(1):119-137.

3.   Brosen K. Some aspects of genetic polymorphism in the biotransformation of antidepressants. *Therapie* 2004; 59(1):5-12.

4.   Yin OQ, Wing YK, Cheung Y, Wang ZJ, Lam SL, Chiu HF, Chow MS. Phenotype-genotype relationship and clinical effects of citalopram in Chinese patients. *J Clin Psychopharmacol* 2006; 26(4):367-372.

5.   Kirchheiner J, Nickchen K, Bauer M, Wong ML, Licinio J, Roots I, Brockmoller J. Pharmacogenetics of antidepressants and antipsychotics: the contribution of allelic variations to the phenotype of drug response. *Mol Psychiatry* 2004; 9(5):442-473.

6.   Murphy GM, Jr., Kremer C, Rodrigues HE, Schatzberg AF. Pharmacogenetics of antidepressant medication intolerance. *Am J Psychiatry* 2003; 160(10):1830-1835.

7.   Suzuki Y, Sawamura K, Someya T. Polymorphisms in the 5-hydroxytryptamine 2A receptor and cytochrome P4502D6 genes synergistically predict fluvoxamine-induced side effects in Japanese depressed patients. *Neuropsychopharmacology* 2006; 31(4):825-831.

8.   Mrazek DA, Smoller JW, de LJ. Incorporating pharmacogenetics into clinical practice: Reality of a new tool in psychiatry. *CNS Spectr* 2006; 11(3 Suppl 3):1-13.

9.   de Leon J, Armstrong SC, Cozza KL. Clinical guidelines for psychiatrists for the use of pharmacogenetic testing for CYP450 2D6 and CYP450 2C19. *Psychosomatics* 2006; 47(1):75-85.

10.   Rush AJ, Fava M, Wisniewski SR, Lavori PW, Trivedi MH, Sackeim HA,

Thase ME, Nierenberg AA, Quitkin FM, Kashner TM. Sequenced treatment

alternatives to relieve depression (STAR*D): rationale and design. *Controlled

Clinical Trials* 2004; 25(1):119-142.

11.   Hiemke C, Hartter S. Pharmacokinetics of selective serotonin reuptake

inhibitors. *Pharmacology & Therapeutics* 2000; 85(1):11-28.

12.   Brosen K, Naranjo CA. Review of pharmacokinetic and pharmacodynamic

interaction studies with citalopram. *European Neuropsychopharmacology* 2001;

11(4):275-283.

13.   Uhr M, Grauer MT. abcb1ab P-glycoprotein is involved in the uptake of

citalopram and trimipramine into the brain of mice. *Journal of Psychiatric Research*

2003; 37(3):179-185.

14.   Hyttel J. Comparative pharmacology of selective serotonin reuptake inhibitors

(SSRIs). *Nord J Psychiatry* 1993; 47(suppl 30):5-12.

15.   Trivedi MH, Rush AJ, Wisniewski SR, Nierenberg AA, Warden D, Ritz L,

Norquist G, Howland RH, Lebowitz B, McGrath PJ, Shores-Wilson K, Biggs MM,

Balasubramani GK, Fava M, Team DS. Evaluation of outcomes with citalopram for

depression using measurement-based care in STAR*D: Implications for clinical

practice. *Am J Psychiatry* 2006; 163(1):28-40.

16.   Kraft JB, Peters EJ, Slager SL, Jenkins GD, Reinalda MS, McGrath PJ,

Hamilton SP. Analysis of association between the serotonin transporter and

antidepressant response in a large clinical sample. *Biol Psychiatry* 2006; advanced

online publication.

17.   Rush AJ, Trivedi MH, Ibrahim HM, Carmody TJ, Arnow B, Klein DN,

Markowitz JC, Ninan PT, Kornstein S, Manber R. The 16-Item quick inventory of depressive symptomatology (QIDS), clinician rating (QIDS-C), and self-report (QIDS-SR): a psychometric evaluation in patients with chronic major depression. *Biol Psychiatry* 2003; 54(5):573-583.

18. Ross DC, Quitkin FM, Klein DF. A typological model for estimation of drug and placebo effects in depression. *J Clin Psychopharmacol* 2002; 22(4):414-418.

19. Quitkin FM, Rabkin JD, Markowitz JM, Stewart JW, McGrath, PJ, Harrison W. Use of pattern analysis to identify true drug response. A replication. *Arch Gen Psychiatry* 1987; 44(3):259-264.

20. McMahon FJ, Buervenich S, Charney D, Lipsky R, Rush AJ, Wilson AF, Sorant AJ, Papanicolaou GJ, Laje G, Fava M, Trivedi MH, Wisniewski SR, Manji H. Variation in the gene encoding the serotonin 2A receptor is associated with outcome of antidepressant treatment. *Am J Hum Genet* 2006; 78(5):804-814.

21. Illmer T, Schuler US, Thiede C, Schwarz UI, Kim RB, Gotthard S, Freund D, Schakel U, Ehninger G, Schaich M. MDR1 gene polymorphisms affect therapy outcome in acute myeloid leukemia patients. *Cancer Res* 2002; 62(17):4955-4962.

22. Hoffmeyer S, Burk O, von RO, Arnold HP, Brockmoller J, Johne A, Cascorbi I, Gerloff T, Roots I, Eichelbaum M, Brinkmann U. Functional polymorphisms of the human multidrug-resistance gene: multiple sequence variations and correlation of one allele with P-glycoprotein expression and activity in vivo. *Proc Natl Acad Sci U S A* 2000; 97(7):3473-3478.

23. Hersberger M, Marti-Jaun J, Rentsch K, Hanseler E. Rapid detection of the CYP2D6*3, CYP2D6*4, and CYP2D6*6 alleles by tetra-primer PCR and of the CYP2D6*5 allele by multiplex long PCR. *Clin Chem* 2000; 46(8 Pt 1):1072-1077.

24. Rodriguez-Antona C, Sayi JG, Gustafsson LL, Bertilsson L, Ingelman-Sundberg M. Phenotype-genotype variability in the human CYP3A locus as assessed

by the probe drug quinine and analyses of variant CYP3A4 alleles. *Biochem Biophys Res Commun* 2005; 338(1):299-305.

25.   Satagopan JM, Venkatraman ES, Begg CB. Two-stage designs for gene-disease association studies with sample size constraints. *Biometrics* 2004; 60(3):589-597.

26.   Schaid DJ, Rowland CM, Tines DE, Jacobson RM, Poland GA. Score tests for association between traits and haplotypes when linkage phase is ambiguous. *Am J Hum Genet* 2002; 70(2):425-434.

27.   Grasmander K, Verwohlt PL, Rietschel M, Dragicevic A, Muller M, Hiemke C, Freymann N, Zobel A, Maier W, Rao ML. Impact of polymorphisms of cytochrome-P450 isoenzymes 2C9, 2C19 and 2D6 on plasma concentrations and clinical effects of antidepressants in a naturalistic clinical setting. *Eur J Clin Pharmacol* 2004; 60(5):329-336.

28.   Mrazek DA. New tool: genotyping makes prescribing safer, more effective. *Curr Psych* 2004; 3(9):11-23.

29.   Rasmussen BB, Brosen K. Is therapeutic drug monitoring a case for optimizing clinical outcome and avoiding interactions of the selective serotonin reuptake inhibitors? *Ther Drug Monit* 2000; 22(2):143-154.

30.   Rudberg I, Hendset M, Uthus LH, Molden E, Refsum H. Heterozygous mutation in CYP2C19 significantly increases the concentration/dose ratio of racemic citalopram and escitalopram (S-citalopram). *Ther Drug Monit* 2006; 28(1):102-105.

31.   Yu BN, Chen GL, He N, Ouyang DS, Chen XP, Liu ZQ, Zhou HH. Pharmacokinetics of citalopram in relation to genetic polymorphism of CYP2C19. *Drug Metab Dispos* 2003; 31(10):1255-1259.

32.   Herrlin K, Yasui-Furukori N, Tybring G, Widen J, Gustafsson LL, Bertilsson L.
Metabolism of citalopram enantiomers in CYP2C19/CYP2D6 phenotyped panels of
healthy Swedes. *British Journal of Clinical Pharmacology* 2003; 56(4):415-421.

33.   Bondolfi G, Chautems C, Rochat B, Bertschy G, Baumann P. Non-response to
citalopram in depressive patients: pharmacokinetic and clinical consequences of a
fluvoxamine augmentation. *Psychopharmacology (Berl)* 1996; 128(4):421-425.

34.   Reis M, Lundmark J, Bengtsson F. Therapeutic drug monitoring of racemic
citalopram: a 5-year experience in Sweden, 1992-1997. *Ther Drug Monit* 2003;
25(2):183-191.

35.   Tang H, Quertermous T, Rodriguez B, Kardia SL, Zhu X, Brown A, Pankow
JS, Province MA, Hunt SC, Boerwinkle E, Schork NJ, Risch NJ. Genetic structure,
self-identified race/ethnicity, and confounding in case-control association studies. *Am
J Hum Genet* 2005; 76(2):268-275.

36.   Tate SK, Depondt C, Sisodiya SM, Cavalleri GL, Schorge S, Soranzo N, Thom
M, Sen A, Shorvon SD, Sander JW, Wood NW, Goldstein DB. Genetic predictors of
the maximum doses patients receive during clinical use of the anti-epileptic drugs
carbamazepine and phenytoin. *PNAS* 2005; 102(15):5507-5512.

CHAPTER 6

WHOLE GENOME ASSOCIATION STUDY OF CITALOPRAM REMISSION

AND TOLERANCE

6.1 Introduction

While candidate gene study designs are often utilized in the investigation of

complex diseases, having *a prioi* knowledge of the causative (or even likely

causative) candidate genes is often difficult for most phenotypes. Indeed,

identification of *new* genes is often the driving force behind complex disease studies.

Gene-agnostic genome-wide linkage studies have been performed for years, but as

discussed in Chapter 1, logistical difficulties arise from collecting families for

pharmacogenetic studies. Recent advances in SNP genotyping technology and

reduction in costs have made whole genome association (WGA) studies feasible (1).

The first reports of WGA studies are just beginning to appear in the literature and

there have been some great success such as the CFH gene and macular degeneration

(2), however, complexities and questions remain regarding the optimal analysis of

WGA data (3). The obvious strength of being able to assay most of the genes in the

human genome is tempered by concerns about multiple testing penalties, population

stratification, and the apparent non-replication of many smaller candidate gene

association studies (4). There is still much debate over the most powerful method for

detecting interacting loci (SNP x SNP), which will be critical for successful mapping

in a common-disease common-variant framework, where individual variants will not

display great increases in risk of having the phenotype. Despite these methodological

considerations, large WGA studies are currently underway such as the Wellcome

Trust Case Control Consortium (WTCCC), which will genotype over 16,000 subjects

170

with various common diseases as well as 3,000 control samples, and the Genetic Association Information Network (GAIN). Both of these projects are consortium-based and have pledged to make their raw genotype and clinical data publicly available shortly after it is generated, allowing other investigators to apply different analytical strategies.

We embarked on a large WGA study using a subset of the STAR*D patient population for which DNA samples were collected, which consists of over 1,900 depressed subjects taking the SSRI citalopram. In order to limit Type I error and reduce overall genotyping costs, we used a two-stage study design (5). In the first stage, we genotyped approximately half of the sample (discovery set, N=967) for 591,158 SNPs distributed across the human genome. The most highly associated SNPs were then genotyped in the second half of the sample (validation set, N=985) to assess if they would replicate the initial association.

Here we report the initial analysis of the WGA data, including descriptions of the genotype data manipulation and quality control checks. Single locus SNP association results are reported for the remission and intolerance phenotypes in the self-identified Caucasian, non-Hispanic subjects, which is the largest racial subgroup. In addition to single locus testing, we also report on the development and testing of multi-SNP clinical decision trees. While none of the putative associations investigated in the second stage replicated their strong initial associations, as discussed below, this is a very preliminary analysis involving the "lowest hanging fruit" and as such, broader, more comprehensive genotyping in the validation sample set needs to be performed. The results of those experiments will be reported in the future elsewhere.

6.2 Methods

6.2.1 STAR*D study population. The study population consisted of the subjects who consented to give DNA from the STAR*D antidepressant trial, as reviewed elsewhere (see Chapter 5). Within each ethnic group, and gender, we randomly split our subjects *a priori* into a discovery and validation sample set (Table 6.1). The entire discovery set was genotyped using the WGA platforms. Due to heterogeneity within our self-identified "White" subjects, as uncovered via the *structure* analysis described below, all analyses were split into three racial subgroups: White, non-Hispanic; White, Hispanic; and African American. Other self-reported race classes were not analyzed.

6.2.2 Discovery set genotyping. A total of four high density SNP panels were used to genotype the discovery set. The Affymetrix 500K array (6) was used (N=500,568 successful SNPs), and genotypes were scored using Affymetrix's BRLMM algorithm (7). In addition, ParAllele's molecular inversion probe (MiP) technology (8) was utilized to genotype a panel of coding region SNPs (cSNPs, N=19,986), a panel of gene-centric SNPs (N=20,127), and a "linker" panel designed to fill in the regions with low coverage on the 500K array (N=50,477). In total, we received successful genotype calls for a total of 591,158 SNPs.

6.2.3 Validation set genotyping. SNPs that were significantly associated in the discovery set with citalopram remission or intolerance in the largest racial subgroup (Non-Hispanic White) were genotyped in the validation set using 5' exonuclease (Taqman) assays. A total of 14 SNPs were genotyped in the validation set (Table 6.2), in an attempt to validate single locus associations and SNP interaction decision trees. We also re-genotyped the discovery set for these SNPs using the Taqman

	Discovery Set			Validation Set		
	Non-Hispanic White	Hispanic White	African American	Non-Hispanic White	Hispanic White	African American
Remitter	336	49	61	263	39	42
Non-Responder	238	61	73	186	33	55
Unclassified	62	13	16	194	52	66
Tolerant	506	91	104	427	60	78
Intolerant	52	7	9	101	26	14
Unclassified	78	25	37	115	38	71

Table 6.1. Sample sizes for the discovery and validation sample sets. Shown are the number of subjects with each phenotype classification for the remission vs. non-responder (top) comparison, and the tolerant vs. intolerant (bottom) comparison. Subjects are divided into discovery and validation sets, and further subdivided by self reported race. Unclassified refers to subjects who did not meet our classification criteria. For the remission phenotype, generally these subjects were not in the study long enough (<4 weeks) to make accurate determination of their response to citalopram. For the intolerance phenotype, the unclassified subjects did not meet the STAR*D algorithm for intolerance or tolerance and were classified as probably intolerant and probably tolerant; these subjects were not used in our analyses.

assays in order to assess the quality of the initial WGA genotyping. For a description of the laboratory methods used for the Taqman assays, see section 4.2.7.

6.2.4 WGA data manipulation and quality control. Raw genotype data files were output to us by Affymetrix in long (samples as columns in the database) form and were converted to wide (SNPs as columns) form in order to perform data analysis. This transposition was accomplished using a custom Perl script kindly provided by Jason Peters ("transpose_rows_columns_NSP_STY.pl").

We removed six samples from the dataset due to low sample call rates (<85%), leaving 633 White non-Hispanic, 121 White Hispanic, and 149 African American samples in the final discovery dataset. Of the 591,158 SNPs that were successfully genotyped, we removed: 282 SNPs which had no chromosomal annotation in dbSNP, 1,129 SNPs that had a call rate less that 85% across the entire discovery set, 1,589 SNPs that were monomorphic across the entire discovery set, and 5,935 SNPs that were duplicated across panels. The remaining SNPs (N=582,223) were used in the analyses described below. In order to be tested for association to citalopram response phenotypes, SNPs were required to conform to Hardy-Weinberg equilibrium (HWE). SNPs with a significant departure from HWE (p<0.00001) were excluded from association analysis. SNPs were tested for departure from HWE within each racial subgroup. Using this threshold, 11,529 SNPs were dropped from analysis in the White, non-Hispanic subgroup. This threshold is conservative, given that our Bonferroni corrected p-value for 582,223 tests at a study-wide alpha of 0.05 would be $p < 8.6 \times 10^{-8}$.

SNP data quality control and descriptive statistics were generated using custom do-files ("WGA_QC.do", "MAF_Analysis.do", "WGA_Spacing.do", written by Eric Peters) and executed in STATA-MP version 9.

Phenotype	Analysis	dbSNP ID	ABI Taqman ID	Gene	Chr.	Chr. position
Remission	single locus	rs4246510	C___3147092_10	-	1	38886987
Remission	single locus	rs6660134	C__30419851_10	-	1	38885739
Remission	single locus	rs10183914	C____157561_10	NFE2L2	2	177923173
Remission	single locus / interaction	rs12033075	C__31226656_10	-	1	53609538
Remission	interaction	rs2514276	C___1747463_10	-	11	90945600
Remission	interaction	rs4821197	C___2520477_10	-	22	32649854
Tolerance	single locus	rs16900795	C__32750710_10	CDH6	5	31297645
Tolerance	single locus	rs828360	C___8945981_10	HTR1E	6	87705285
Tolerance	single locus	rs6489035	C__29408252_10	-	12	124928948
Tolerance	single locus	rs7145321	C___1815889_10	-	14	65507316
Tolerance	single locus	rs1367841	C___2050336_10	CPEB1	15	81107680
Tolerance	interaction	rs4512110	C__28976342_10	COL4A3BP	5	74791977
Tolerance	interaction	rs2648849	C__16055367_10	-	8	129251833
Tolerance	interaction	rs17600619	C__33544364_10	-	13	58057924

Table 6.2. Follow-up SNPs genotyped in the validation sample set. Four single locus associations were tested for the remission phenotype comparison, five were tested for the intolerance phenotype comparison. Three SNPs in each phenotype comparison were tested in the interaction analysis. Shown are the dbSNP IDs for the 14 SNPs, as well as the ABI Taqman assay ID. Chromosome, chromosome position, and gene annotation (if applicable) are from NCBI build 35.

6.2.5 LD analysis. In order to assay the amount of redundancy in the SNP genotype data, SNP binning based on pairwise r^2 values was performed. Within each racial subgroup (White, non-Hispanic, White Hispanic, and African American), pairwise r^2 for each SNP with all other SNPs within a 1 megabase sliding window was calculated. This process was repeated for all the SNPs in the WGA panel. Data was then complied, any redundancy was removed, and the number of proxy SNPs at several r^2 thresholds was calculated. This was performed using custom do-files ("LD_R2_binning.do" and "Appending_LD_bins.do", written by Eric Peters) and executed in STATA-MP version 9.

6.2.6 *Structure* analysis. In order to assess the levels of genetic heterogeneity in the sample, the MCMC method of Pritchard et al was performed, as implemented in *Structure* version 2.0 (9). Using the discovery sample set and 500 random SNPs from the WGA data from across the genome, the algorithm was run using 100,000 burn-ins followed by 1,000,000 iterations. Several runs were performed assuming from 1 to 4 underlying subpopulations ("K"), and results for each "K" were stable in terms of estimates of alpha, Fst, and proportion ancestry ("Q") for each individual, indicating the algorithm had not inadvertently settled at a local maximum. However, given that the validation sample set was genotyped for a very limited number of markers, a corresponding analysis could not be performed in that group.

6.2.7 Single locus analysis. In this report, we focused all the association analyses on the largest racial subgroup, self-identified non-Hispanic White subjects. We investigated two clinical phenotypes, citalopram remission (defined as a final QIDS score of less than 6), and intolerance to citalopram (defined using clinical exit and GRSEB data). Both of these phenotypes have been described in detail previously for this study population (see section 5.2.2). We used a custom do-file ("single_locus_analysis.do", written by Eric Peters and incorporating the genass2.ado script kindly provided by Dr. Neil Shephard) to test each SNP in the WGA panel for association to the two phenotypes within the White non-Hispanic subgroup in the discovery set. Only SNPs that passed the QC filters described above were used in the association analysis. Given that we do not know the mode of inheritance *a priori*, we used a genotypic model (data coded as: AA, Aa, aa), and Fisher's exact test to investigate single locus associations. Dominant (minor allele carrier versus non-carrier) odds ratios for each SNP were also calculated.

The selection of our statistical threshold for which SNPs to genotype in the validation sample set was based on the capacity to genotype these samples in the lab for minimal costs. As such, we only sought to investigate the most highly associated SNPs. Our threshold was a p-value of less than 1×10^{-5} using the genotypic model in the discovery set, which yielded a reasonable number of SNPs to follow up using singleplex genotyping assays. We then required these follow-up SNPs to have a $p<0.05$ in the validation sample set in order to declare study-wide significance.

6.2.8 Interactions. In order to test for SNP x SNP interactions, as well as interactions between SNPs and clinical covariates, we developed decision trees using the discovery dataset and tested them using the validation sample set. Decisions trees were constructed for both phenotype comparisons in the White, non-Hispanic subgroup. The entire genotype data of the discovery set, along with age, gender, marital status, depression subtype, recurrence, and severity at baseline were all included in the model. The decision tree was built using the most parsimonious split at each node, defined as the division of the data based on a single variable's value that creates the two most distinct subnodes, as measured by the frequency of the phenotype (e.g., remission) within those subnodes. The data is split in this way until no further statistically significant splits can be made. Genotypic splits were allowed using either recessive or dominant models. Since this is the model generation step, we only required a Bonferroni corrected p<0.1 to declare a split statistically significant.

We used the validation data set to empirically assess the clinical significance of the decision trees. In order to utilize these trees, a subject is "run" through the model (starting at the top, and continuing in whichever direction their genotype dictates), until a terminal node is reached. That subject's predicted probability of having the phenotype in question is equal to the frequency of that phenotype in the same terminal node using the discovery set data. We rounded the subject's phenotype probability to a dichotomous variable (e.g., 1 or 0) and assessed the significance of the decision trees using standard diagnostic test metrics. Alternatively, logistic regression with the actual outcome as the dependent variable and the subject's phenotype probability (from the decision tree) as the independent variable was used to assess the statistical significance of the decision trees. Interaction analyses were performed in HelixTree and STATA-MP version 9.

6.3 Results

6.3.1 WGA data descriptions and QC. A total of 582,223 unique SNPs passed our QC filters that are described in the methods section. Overall, these SNPs had a very high call rate (mean 99.1%, standard deviation 1.7%). There were 5,935 SNPs that were assayed across multiple panels. These duplicated SNPs had a genotype concordance of 99.59% (21,740 discordant genotypes out of 5,254,488 possible comparisons).

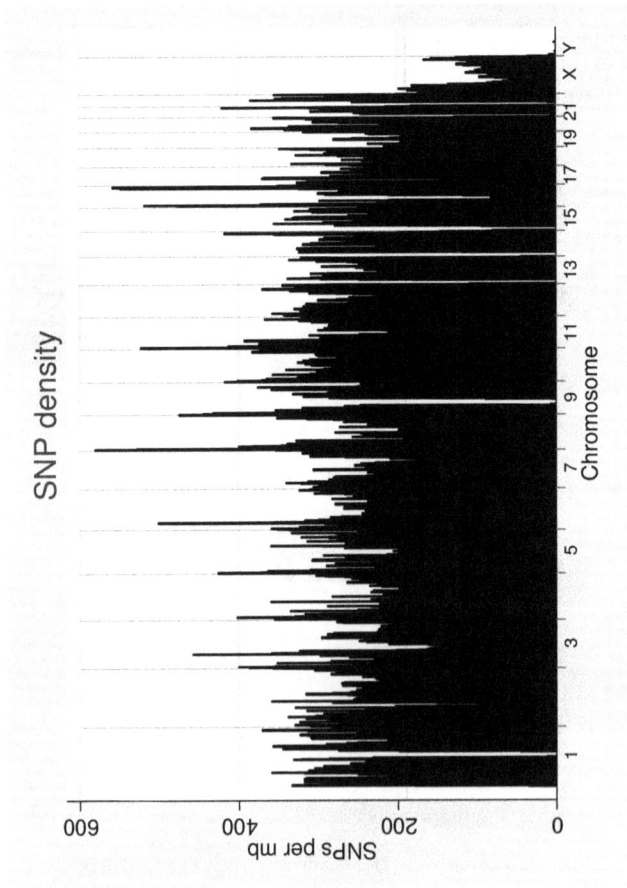

SNP density

Figure 6.1

179

Figure 6.1. SNP marker density across the genome. Shown is the SNP density (y-axis, in SNPs per megabase) versus physical position across the genome, which is shown on the x-axis (chromosome 1 to Y, left to right). Large gaps seen are centromeric and telomeric portions of the chromosomes, where hybridization-based SNP assays do not work. Average density is shown by horizontal dashed line, approximately 190 SNPs per megabase.

SNPs were not uniformly distributed across the entire genome. Large gaps exist in centromeric and telomeric regions of some chromosomes, as seen in Figure 6.1. This is due to technical difficulties that arise from assaying those regions which are abundant in repetitive DNA sequences. On average, there were approximately 190 SNPs assayed per megabase of sequence. Assay coverage was markedly lower on the X and Y chromosomes. On average there was a marker every 4.9 kb (median 2.3 kb), though the distribution of intermarker distances is skewed due to a small number of very large gaps (Figure 6.2).

Marker minor allele distribution varied between racial subgroups. The white non-Hispanics subgroup had fewer SNPs with a minor allele frequency greater than 5% than the African American subgroup (447,696 and 502,194, respectively, see Figure 6.3). Large differences in allele frequencies for individual SNPs were observed between the White non-Hispanic and African American subgroups (Figure 6.4). This highlights the potential for confounding due to genetic structure, which we hope to avoid by testing for association within self-identified racial subgroups.

6.3.2 *Structure* analysis. Population stratification can lead to confounding in case-control association studies. We ran a *Structure* analysis on the discovery sample set using 500 random SNPs from across the genome (Figure 6.5). Results indicated that a model with three genetic subgroups (i.e., K=3) was the best fit for the data. Clear distinction was seen between the self-reported African American and White samples, and the third genetic subpopulation correlated well with Hispanic ancestry. Due to the fact that we did not genotype enough markers in the validation set for a similar *structure* analysis, we used self-reported racial and ethnic status as a proxy for genetically determined ancestry. Thus, all analyses presented here are within these subgroups (non-Hispanic White, Hispanic White, African American), unless

181

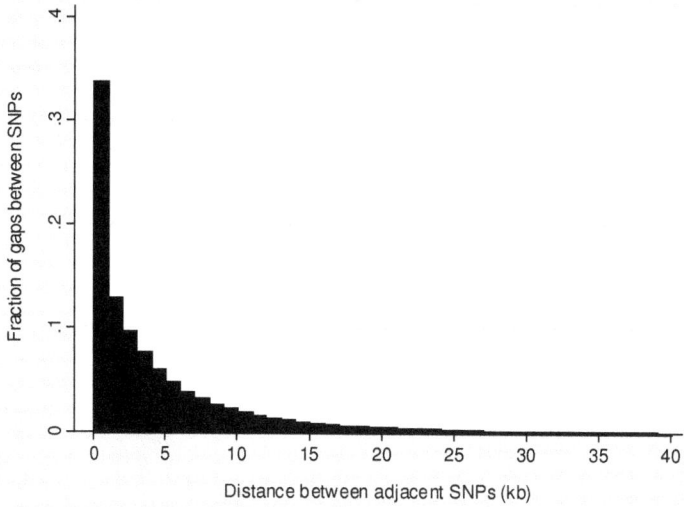

Figure 6.2. Hisotgram of inter-marker distances. Shown is the distance between adjacent SNPs (kb) on the x-axis (in 1 kb bins), and the proportion of gaps with that given distance (y-axis). The distribution is skewed (average gap = 4.9 kb, median = 2.3 kb) due to a small number of very large gaps.

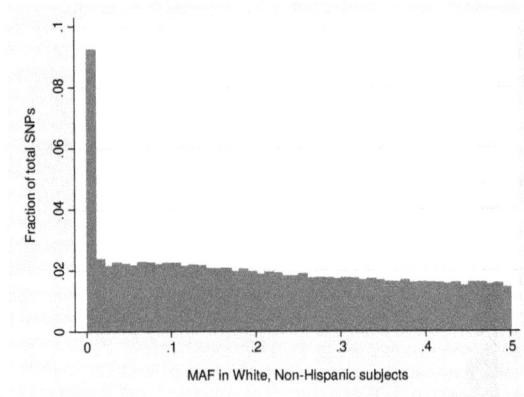

a)

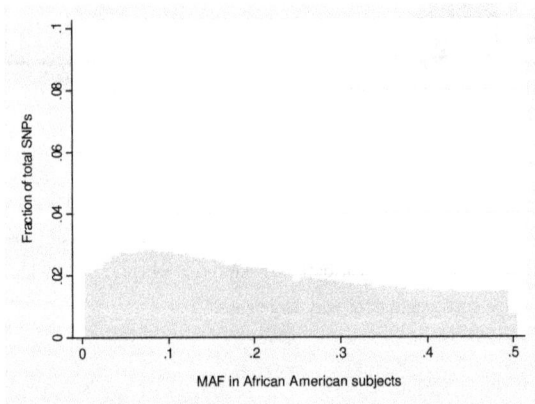

b)

Figure 6.3. Histogram of SNPs by minor allele frequencies (MAF) in each racial subgroup. On the x-axis is the SNP MAF (in 1% bins), with each bin's proportion of the total SNPs shown on the y-axis. a) Results for the non-Hispanic White subgroup. Note the skewed distribution, with almost 10% of the SNPs having a MAF of 1% or less. Only 77% of the total markers had a MAF greater than 5%. b.) Results for the African American subgroup. The distribution is almost flat, with 86% of the total markers having a greater than 5% MAF.

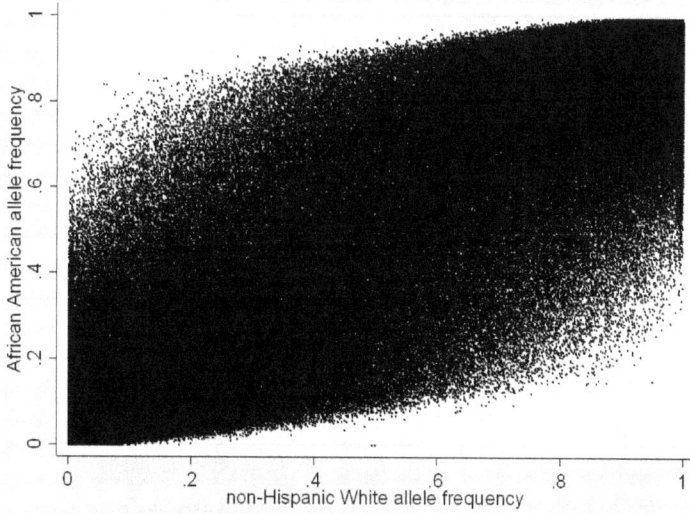

Figure 6.4. Scatterplot of SNP allele frequency by racial subgroup. Each of the discovery set genotypes is represented as a single point, with African American allele frequency on the y-axis and non-Hispanic White allele frequency on the x-axis.

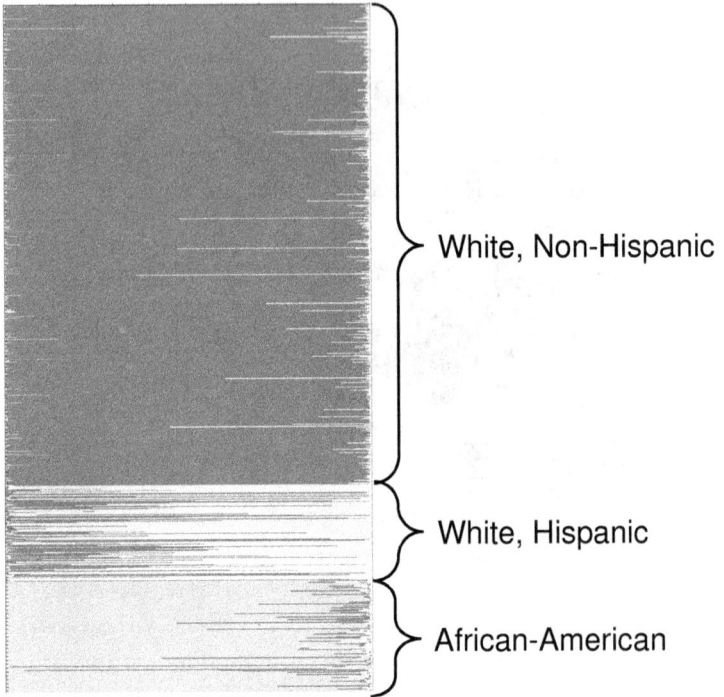

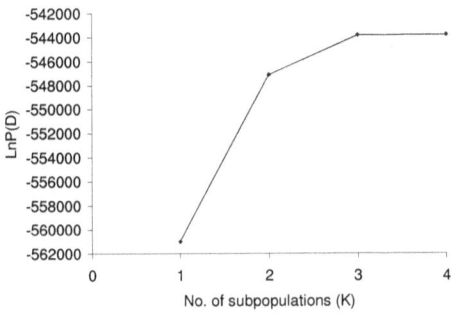

Figure 6.5

185

Figure 6.5. Results of *Structure* analysis using 500 random SNPs in the discovery sample set. Top plot shows the percent identity (Q) from the three historical subpopulations for each subject. Subjects are ordered based on self-reported race, as shown to the right of the *Structure* plot. Also shown is a graph of the posterior probability of the model at various numbers of historical subpopulations (K). As can be seen, the addition of a 4th subpopulation does not significantly strengthen the model fit, thus a K=3 was used.

otherwise noted.

6.3.3 LD analysis. Not surprisingly, given the marker density in this study, there was a great amount of LD between the SNPs on our WGA panels. As expected based on population history, the African American subgroup showed less LD on average than the non-Hispanic White subgroup (Figure 6.6). For instance, for common SNPs (MAF>5%) within 5 kb of each other, the average pairwise r^2 was 0.4 in the non-Hispanic White subgroup, and 0.27 in the African American subgroup. Average LD decayed relatively uniformly with distance, but as can be seen below, there were clusters of SNPs with locally high levels of LD.

In order to get a sense of the redundancy of the genotype data, which is an important consideration in determining the number of independent tests performed, we ran an r^2 threshold binning approach on the common SNPs in the WGA panels (Figure 6.7a). Using a sliding window of 1mb around the target SNP, the number of proxy SNPs was determined using various thresholds of r^2. These analyses revealed significant redundancy in the SNPs genotyped. In the non-Hispanic White subgroup, using an $r^2=1$ threshold, which means the genotype of one SNP perfectly predicts the genotype of another SNP in all cases, over 9% of the SNPs have at least one perfect proxy. At a reduced, but still conservative, threshold of $r^2=0.95$, over 30% of the SNPs have at least one very good proxy in the dataset. In the African American subgroup, redundancy was still high, though less than in the non-Hispanic Whites (Figure 6.7b).

6.3.4 Single locus association – discovery set. We performed two phenotype comparisons in our non-Hispanic White subjects; remitters versus non-remitters, and citalopram intolerant versus tolerant. The results for all the SNPs across the genome for the remission phenotype are shown in Figure 6.8. While no SNP was significant

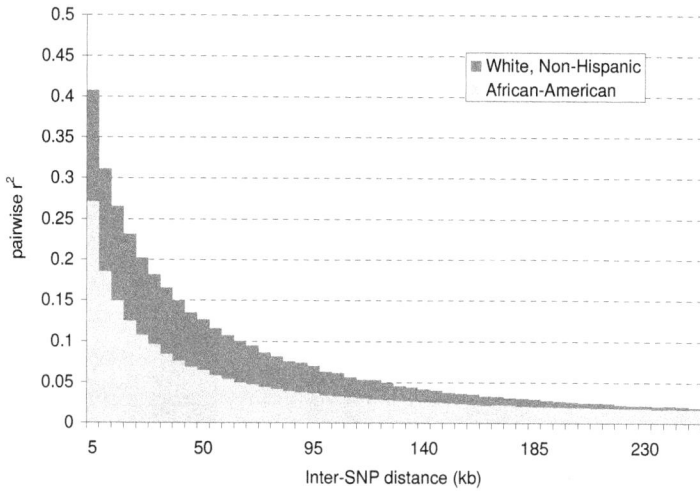

Figure 6.6. Average pairwise r² between SNPs by intermarker distance. Distance between SNPs is shown on the x-axis, in 5 kb intervals. Average pairwise r² for all SNP pairs with intermarker distances within that interval is shown on the y-axis. Results for the non-Hispanic White subgroup are shown in red, African American results are in green. Only common SNPs (>5% MAF) were used in this analysis.

a)

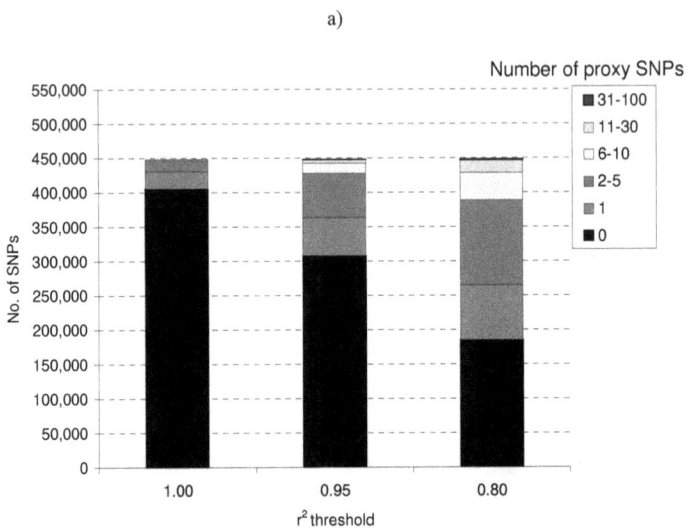

b)

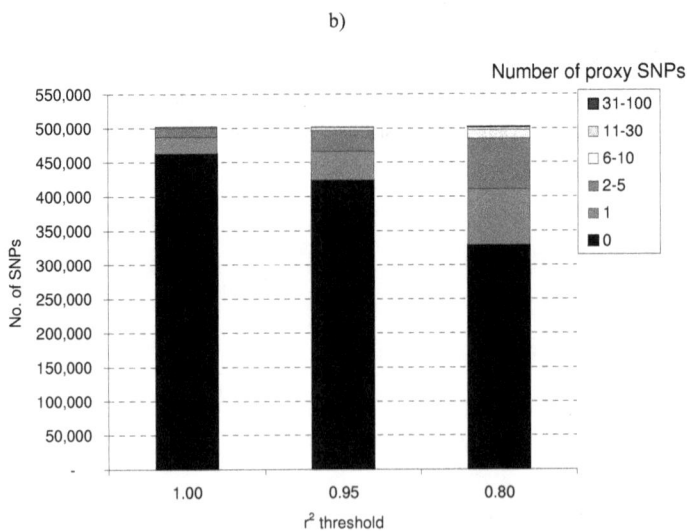

Figure 6.7

Figure 6.7. Redundancy of common SNPs at various r^2 thresholds in each racial subgroup. All common SNPs (>5% MAF) are shown on the y-axis. Using a sliding window of 1mb around the target SNP, the number of proxy SNPs (SNPs in LD above the threshold) for each SNP was determined using an r^2 threshold of 1, 0.95 and 0.8 (x-axis). a) Results for the non-Hispanic White subgroup. b) Results for the African American subgroup.

using a Bonferroni corrected threshold ($p < 8.6 \times 10^{-8}$), four SNPs met our threshold ($p < 1 \times 10^{-5}$) for follow-up in the validation sample set. Dominant odds ratios for these SNPs, transformed to >1, ranged from 2 - 3.15 (Table 6.3). None of these variants were also nominally ($p<0.05$) associated in our other two racial subgroups. Quantile-Quantile (QQ) plots for this phenotype comparison showed no gross inflation of the chi-squared statistics (Figure 6.9). Systematic inflation can be indicative of confounding due to population stratification or other factors.

The results for the intolerance phenotype are shown in Figure 6.10. Again, no SNPs met a strict Bonferroni corrected threshold, however five SNPs met our threshold for follow-up in the validation sample set, with dominant ORs, transformed to >1, ranging from 1.5 to 12.6 (Table 6.4). None of the SNPs were also nominally associated ($p<0.05$) with intolerance in our other two racial subgroups. QQ plots for this phenotype showed an inflation of the chi-squared statistics (Figure 6.11). While this inflation may be driven by unaccounted for population stratification in our non-Hispanic White subgroup, results of analyzing the entire discovery set, regardless of self-identified race, did not seem to increase the inflation of the chi-squared. Thus, the initial result may be due to the fact that the intolerance phenotype is rare (~9% in the discovery set) and we have several rare SNPs in the panels, thus comparing our results to the standard chi-squared distribution may not be appropriate assumption.

6.3.5 Single locus association – validation set. In order to verify the genotype data we received from our Affymetrix panels was accurate through use of an alterative genotyping method (e.g., Taqman), we genotyped the discovery set as well as the validation set in the second phase of the study. For the remission phenotype, genotype data for three of the four SNPs had high concordance with the Affymetrix

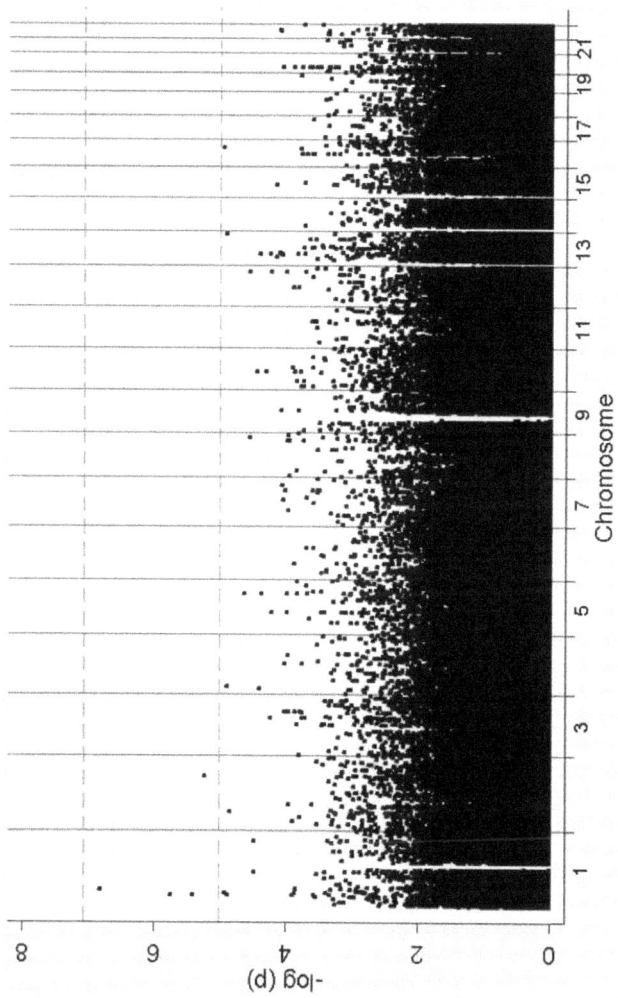

Figure 6.8.

Figure 6.8. Single locus association results in the discovery sample set for the remission phenotype in the non-Hispanic White subgroup. Each point represents a single SNP. The negative log of the p-value for association is shown on the y-axis, and the variants are in order across the genome from chromosome 1-22 on the x-axis. Chromosome X and Y are not shown, but no significant results were obtained on those chromosomes. The dashed line at 1×10^{-7} is approximately the threshold for Bonferroni corrected significance (no SNPs meet this criteria). The dashed line at 1×10^{-5} represents our criteria for testing the association in the validation sample set (four SNPs).

dbSNP ID	Discovery set			
	Remit	NR	p-value	OR (95% CI)
rs4246510	0.39	0.53	3.9E-06	0.39 (0.26, 0.59)
rs6660134	0.42	0.58	1.8E-06	0.40 (0.26, 0.60)
rs12033075	0.16	0.06	1.5E-07	3.15 (1.97, 5.14)
rs10183914	0.35	0.40	6.0E-06	0.50 (0.35, 0.72)

Table 6.3. The most highly associated SNPs for the remission phenotype in the non-Hispanic White subgroup in the discovery set. Shown are the minor allele frequencies in the remitters ("Remit") and non-responders ("NR"). The p-value for association is shown, as well as the odds ratio (OR) and 95% confidence intervals. ORs were calculated using a dominant model (minor allele carrier vs. non-carrier).

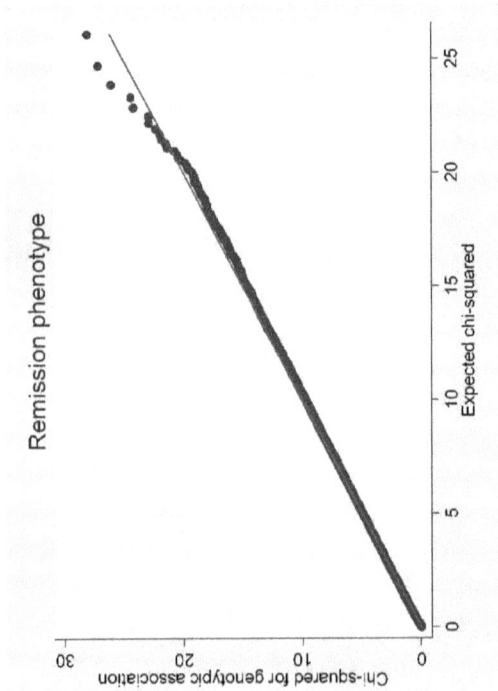

Figure 6.9. Quantile-Quantile (QQ) plots of single locus associations for the remission phenotype in the non-Hispanic White subgroup. The quantiles for the expected chi-squared distribution are shown on the x-axis, and the quantiles for the actual chi-squared distribution are shown on the y-axis. The distribution appears to follow unity (line at 45° from origin) well, indicating that gross inflation of the chi-squared (due to stratification or other reasons) is not present. The four follow up SNPs are seen at the very right-most portion of the plot. While these are above the unity line, the majority of the data is consistent with what one would expect by chance.

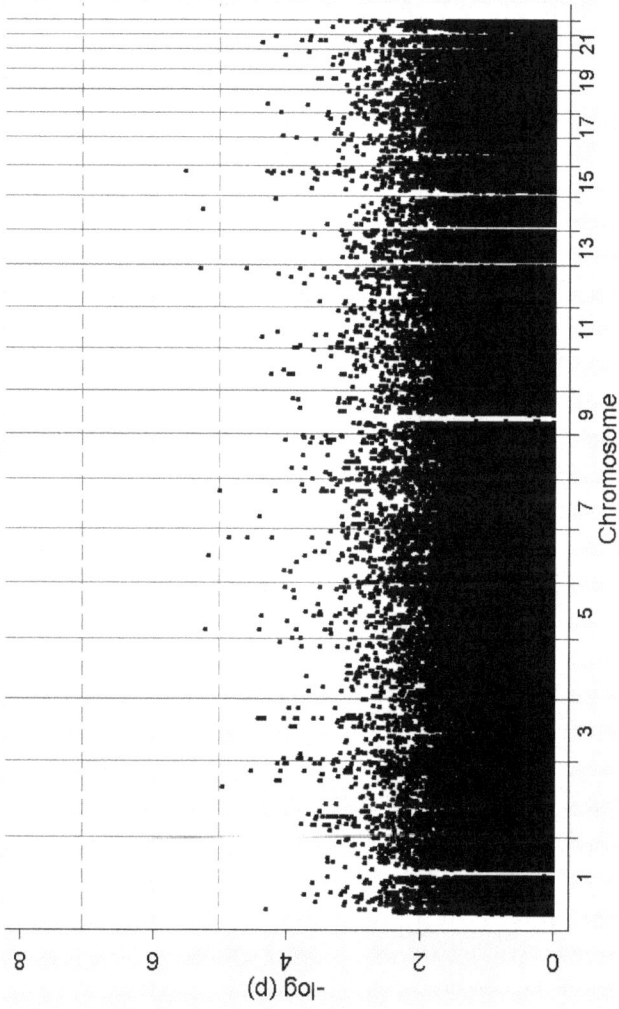

Figure 6.10.

Figure 6.10. Single locus association results in the discovery sample set for the intolerance phenotype in the non-Hispanic White subgroup. Each point represents a single SNP. The negative log of the p-value for association is shown on the y-axis, and the variants are in order across the genome from chromosome 1-22 on the x-axis. Chromosomes X and Y are not shown, but no significant results were obtained on those chromosomes. The dashed line at 1×10^{-7} is approximately the threshold for Bonferroni corrected significance (no SNPs meet this criteria). The dashed line at 1×10^{-5} represents our criteria for testing the association in the validation sample set (five SNPs).

	Discovery set			
dbSNP ID	Intolerant	Tolerant	p-value	OR (95% CI)
rs16900795	0.16	0.04	6.30E-06	0.17 (0.08, 0.37)
rs828360	0.02	0.18	6.92E-06	12.69 (3.26, 108.64)
rs6489035	0.28	0.53	5.18E-06	3.61 (1.93, 6.75)
rs7145321	0.37	0.22	5.67E-06	0.66 (0.36, 1.22)
rs1367841	0.56	0.33	3.11E-06	0.16 (0.06, 0.39)

Table 6.4. The most highly associated SNPs for the intolerance phenotype in the non-Hispanic White subgroup in the discovery set. Shown are the minor allele frequencies in the citalopram tolerant and intolerant subjects. The p-value for association is shown, as well as the odds ratio (OR) and 95% confidence intervals. ORs were calculated using a dominant model (minor allele carrier vs. non-carrier).

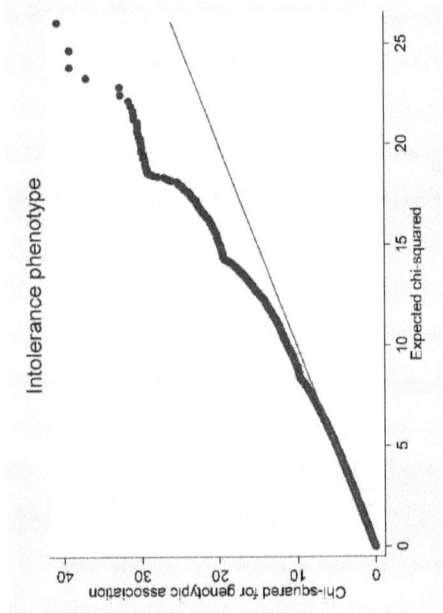

Figure 6.11. Quantile-Quantile (QQ) plots of single locus associations for the intolerance phenotype in the non-Hispanic White subgroup. The quantiles for the expected chi-squared distribution are shown on the x-axis, and the quantiles for the actual chi-squared distribution are shown on the y-axis. The distribution does not follow unity (line at 45° from origin) well, indicating that gross inflation of the chi-squared (due to stratification or other reasons) is present. The reason for this is unknown, but may be due to the rareness of the intolerance phenotype (and several SNPs) and thus the inappropriateness of comparing our results to the standard chi-squared distribution. The five follow-up SNPs are seen at the very right-most portion of the plot.

genotype calls (99.9%). For one SNP (rs4246510), 31 subjects with homozygous

genotypes in the Affymetrix data had heterozygous genotypes using the Taqman

assay, which appear unambiguous (Figure 6.12). Furthermore, by adjusting the

Affymetrix genotype calls in this way SNP rs4246510 has near perfect LD with SNP

rs6660134, which is less than 2 kb away. Indeed these two SNPs are in perfect LD

(e.g., r^2=1) in HapMap data from Caucasian individuals. None of these four SNPs

yielded a significant association to remission in the validation sample (p<0.05), using

the same genotypic model and data coding format as in the discovery set analysis

(Table 6.5).

The genotype concordance between the Affymetrix and Taqman calls was

high (99.8%) for all of the SNPs that were selected for follow-up using the citalopram

intolerance phenotype. Interestingly, one SNP (rs6489035) showed four distinct

clusters on the Taqman raw data plot as opposed to the expected three clusters (Figure

6.13). Subjects that were in the intermediate cluster were scored as missing in our

Taqman data for the validation sample set, while they were generally scored as

heterozygotes in the Affymetrix data. The intermediate fourth cluster accounted for

approximately 6% of subjects. Distinct extra clusters can be caused by repeated DNA

segments or variation in DNA copy number. None of these five SNPs showed

significant association (p<0.05) to intolerance in the validation sample set using the

same analytic methods as in the discovery set analysis (Table 6.6). A single SNP

(rs7145321), had a trend (p<0.06) towards significance in the validation sample set

and the effect had the same directionality as the one observed in the discovery set.

6.3.6 Interaction analysis – discovery set. Multi-node decision trees were

generated for each phenotypic comparison, as described in detail in section 6.2.8.

Briefly, the discovery population is "split" based on the most parsimonious SNP (i.e.,

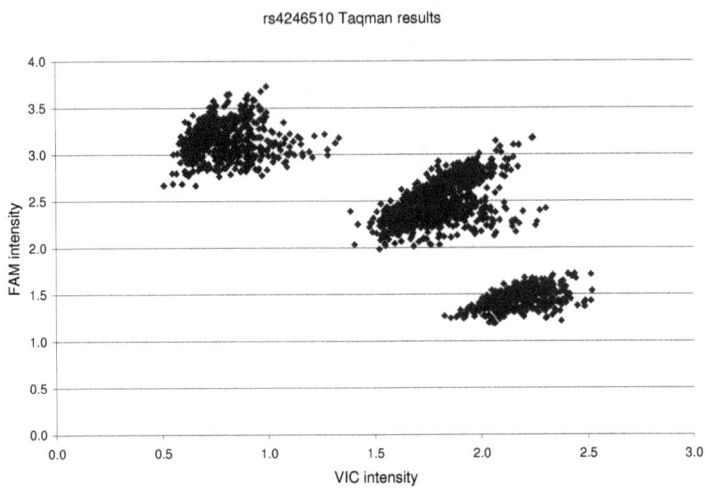

rs4246510 Taqman results

Figure 6.12. Taqman results for SNP rs4246510 across the entire STAR*D sample set. VIC and FAM label intensities are on the x- and y-axis, respectively. Results appear unambiguous, though 31 samples, called via Taqman as heterozygotes, were called homzygotes (FAM) in the Affymetrix data.

	Validation set			
dbSNP ID	Remit	NR	p-value	OR (95% CI)
rs4246510	0.44	0.49	0.42	0.77 (0.49, 1.19)
rs6660134	0.45	0.50	0.32	0.74 (0.47, 1.15)
rs12033075	0.12	0.14	0.57	0.85 (0.53, 1.36)
rs10183914	0.34	0.36	0.81	0.98 (0.65, 1.46)

	Overall			
dbSNP ID	Remit	NR	p-value	OR (95% CI)
rs4246510	0.41	0.51	2.4E-05	0.53 (0.39, 0.71)
rs6660134	0.42	0.52	3.9E-05	0.54 (0.40, 0.72)
rs12033075	0.14	0.09	0.004	1.68 (1.22, 2.32)
rs10183914	0.35	0.38	0.002	0.68 (0.52, 0.89)

Table 6.5. Single locus association results for the remission phenotype follow-up SNPs in the validation sample set. Shown at the top are the results for the validation sample set, and below it are the results for the overall sample (joint analysis). Shown are the minor allele frequencies in the remitters ("Remit") and non-responders ("NR"). The p-value for association is shown, as well as the odds ratio (OR) and 95% confidence intervals. ORs were calculated using a dominant model (minor allele carrier vs. non-carrier). None of these SNPs were significantly associated (p<0.05) in the validation sample set.

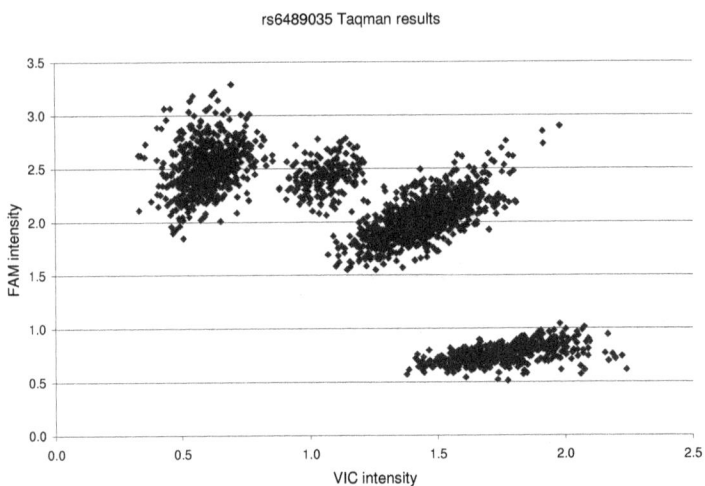

rs6489035 Taqman results

Figure 6.13. Taqman results for SNP rs6489035 across the entire STAR*D sample set. VIC and FAM label intensities are on the x- and y-axis, respectively. Clearly visible is an intermediate fourth cluster, which we coded as "missing" in our Taqman data but was scored as heterozygous in the Affymetrix data. The reason for this fourth cluster is unknown, though it could be caused by structural variation or mis-priming of the probe to related sequence.

the SNP that produces the most differentiated sub-nodes). This process is repeated until no more significant splits can be made. The remission phenotype comparison yielded a tree incorporating three SNPs (Figure 6.14). One of these SNPs, rs12033075, was also significantly associated in the discovery set in our single locus testing above. This final tree predicted the remission status correctly for 395 out of 571 subjects (69%) in the discovery ("training") data set (Table 6.7). The decision tree for the intolerance phenotype included three SNPs (Figure 6.15). This tree was able to correctly predict intolerance status in 514 out of 555 (92%) subjects in the discovery set (Table 6.8).

6.3.7 Interaction analysis – validation set. Concordance between Affymetrix and Taqman genotype calls was high (99.8%) for the six SNPs used in the remission and intolerance decision tree. For the remission phenotype comparison, using the validation sample set genotype data and the predicted probabilities of the terminal nodes from the training set, the decision tree correctly predicted only 227 out of 441 (52%) subject's remission status (Table 6.7). The results were similarly non-significant for the intolerance decision tree, with only 415 out of 522 (80%) of the validation sample subject's intolerance status predicted correctly (Table 6.8). Thus, the decision trees constructed were not prognostic for either remission or intolerance, and likely over-fit the data in the discovery set. Furthermore, neither decision tree yielded quantitative predictions that were significantly associated ($p<0.05$) with the true dichotomous phenotype status via logistic regression (results not shown).

6.4 Discussion

Association studies involving this density of markers present unique analytical and computational challenges. In our study, we pursued a limited number (N=9) of

dbSNP ID	Validation set			
	Intolerant	Tolerant	p-value	OR (95% CI)
rs16900795	0.06	0.04	0.27	0.70 (0.33, 1.60)
rs828360	0.16	0.15	0.75	0.97 (0.59, 1.65)
rs6489035	0.55	0.47	0.15	0.72 (0.40, 1.25)
rs7145321	0.26	0.21	0.06	0.88 (0.55, 1.40)
rs1367841	0.34	0.37	0.11	1.43 (0.90, 2.27)

dbSNP ID	Overall			
	Intolerant	Tolerant	p-value	OR (95% CI)
rs16900795	0.09	0.04	0.0009	0.39 (0.23, 0.66)
rs828360	0.11	0.17	0.01	1.79 (1.16, 2.84)
rs6489035	0.45	0.50	0.22	1.40 (0.94, 2.08)
rs7145321	0.30	0.21	2.03E-06	0.78 (0.54, 1.13)
rs1367841	0.41	0.35	0.09	0.77 (0.53, 1.11)

Table 6.6. Single locus association results for the intolerance phenotype follow-up SNPs in the validation sample set. At the top are the results for the validation sample set, and below it are the results for the overall sample (joint analysis). Shown are the minor allele frequencies in citalopram tolerant and intolerant subjects. The p-value for association is shown, as well as the odds ratio (OR) and 95% confidence intervals. ORs were calculated using a dominant model (minor allele carrier vs. non-carrier). None of these SNPs were significantly associated (p<0.05) in the validation sample set, though a single SNP (rs7145321) was close, with a p=0.06 in the validation set.

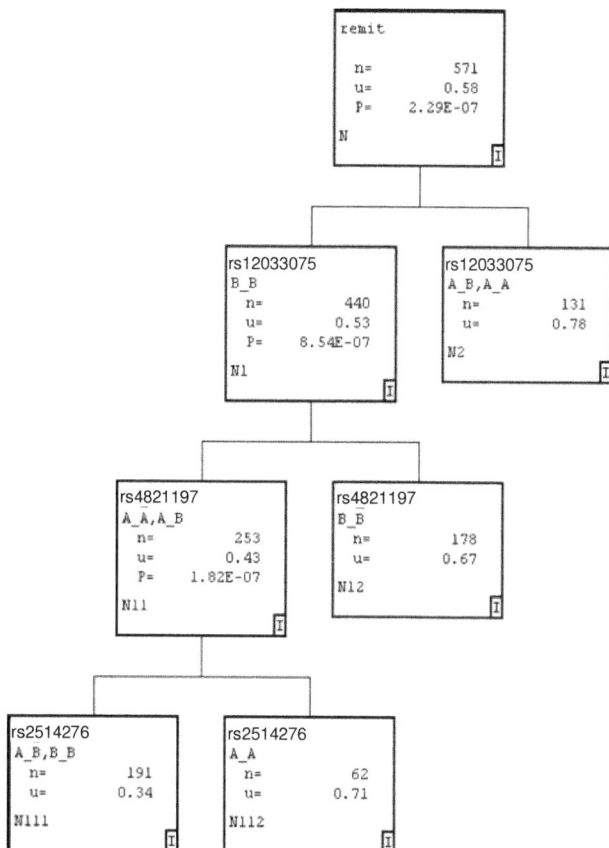

Figure 6.14. Decision tree for the remission phenotype in the non-Hispanic White discovery sample set. The node at the top of this tree contains all the subjects ("n"), the percentage in that node that are remitters ("u"), and the unadjusted p-value for the first split of the sample. The first split (rs12033075) divides the sample into those carrying the "B_B" genotype and those that do not. Partitioning of the sample continues with two additional SNPs.

	Discovery set	

| | Tree prediciton | |
Actual	Remit	NR
Remit	269	65
NR	111	126

Sensitivity: 80.5%
Specificity: 53.2%
Positive predictive value: 70.8%
Negative predictive value: 66.0%
Correctly predicts 395 / 571 (69.2%)

	Validation set	

| | Tree prediciton | |
Actual	Remit	NR
Remit	164	96
NR	118	63

Sensitivity: 63.1%
Specificity: 34.8%
Positive predictive value: 58.2%
Negative predictive value: 39.6%
Correctly predicts 227 / 441 (51.5%)

Table 6.7. Decision tree predictions for the remission phenotype in the discovery and validation sample sets. Shown at top are the predictions of the decision tree and the actual phenotype in the discovery sample set (Remit – remitters, NR – non-responders). The bottom table shows the predictions and actual phenotypes in the validation sample set. Sensitivity (percent of remitters predicted to be remitters), specificity (percent of non-responders predicted to be non-responders), positive predictive value (percent of predicted remitters that are actual remitters), and negative predictive value (percent of predicted non-responders that are actual non-responders) are also displayed.

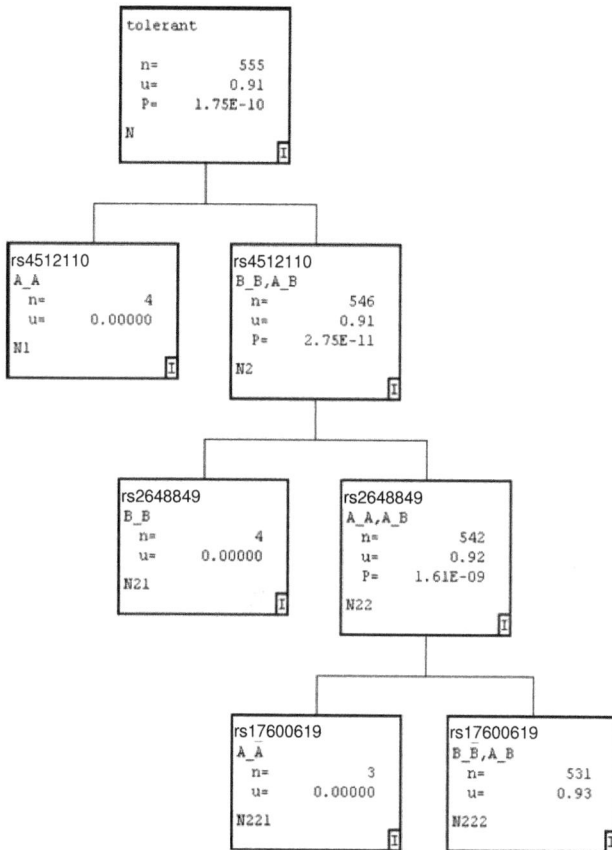

Figure 6.15. Decision tree for the intolerance phenotype in the non-Hispanic White discovery sample set. The node at the top of this tree contains all the subjects ("n"), the percentage in that node that are tolerant to citalopram ("u"), and the unadjusted p-value for the first split of the sample. The first split (rs4512110) divides the sample into those carrying the "A_A" genotype and those that do not. Partitioning of the sample continues with two additional SNPs.

	Discovery set	
	Tree prediciton	
Actual	Intolerant	Tolerant
Intolerant	11	41
Tolerant	0	503

Sensitivity: 21.2%
Specificity: 100%
Positive predictive value: 100%
Negative predictive value: 92.5%
Correctly predicts 514 out of 555 (92.6%)

	Validation set	
	Tree prediciton	
Actual	Intolerant	Tolerant
Intolerant	2	97
Tolerant	10	413

Sensitivity: 2.0%
Specificity: 97.6%
Positive predictive value: 16.7%
Negative predictive value: 81.0%
Correctly predicts 415 out of 522 (79.5%)

Table 6.8. Decision tree predictions for the intolerance phenotype in the discovery and validation sample sets. Shown at top are the predictions of the decision tree and the actual phenotype in the discovery sample set. The bottom table shows the predictions and actual phenotypes in the validation sample set. Sensitivity (percent of intolerant predicted to be intolerant), specificity (percent of tolerant predicted to be tolerant), positive predictive value (percent of predicted intolerant that are actually intolerant), and negative predictive value (percent of predicted tolerant that are actually tolerant) are also displayed.

single locus associations in our validation sample set, none of which replicated (p<0.05) the initial association for either phenotype comparison. One SNP, rs7145321, trended towards significance (p<0.06) in the validation sample set for the intolerance phenotype, in the same directionality of association as seen in the discovery sample set. While it did not meet our criteria for study-wide significance, this variant (which is greater than 200 kb from any known gene) deserves follow-up testing in other study populations taking SSRIs. It has been argued that a joint analysis of the combined discovery and validation sample sets is more powerful than the two-stage replication strategy (10). However, given the low number of SNPs that we chose to replicate here, it is unclear what the most statistically powerful strategy is. We chose a replication based strategy as we were chiefly interested in the ability of the putatively associated SNPs to consistently show association in different populations. In order for these SNPs to be used in clinical decision making, replication in different populations is essential – non-replication of putative associations is a sobering reality that is common with complex genetic phenotypes. In addition to our single locus testing, we also genotyped five additional SNPs in the validation sample set in an attempt to replicate multi-SNP decision trees constructed for each phenotype using the discovery dataset. These decision trees did not have useful predictive power in the validation sample set.

Given that we had an adequate sample size to replicate the initial associations in the validation set, the reason for the lack of replication is unclear, though there could be several underlying causes. In order to limit Type I error in the screening stage and to limit the amount of replication SNPs to be genotyped in-house with singleplex assays, we only attempted to replicate SNPs that were associated above a conservative p-value threshold ($p<1\times10^{-5}$). However, none of the associations in either phenotype comparison would survive a Bonferroni correction for multiple comparisons, so there is a reasonable risk that these are false-positive signals in the discovery dataset. Unfortunately, it's unclear how many independent tests were performed and thus require adjustment, given the high levels of LD seen in the data. Population stratification could also be underlying the lack of replication. We attempted to control for population stratification using self-reported race, including Hispanic ancestry, as a proxy for genetic ancestry. This strategy was guided by a *Structure* analysis using 500 SNPs in the discovery population dataset. Ideally, we would be able to cluster the subjects for analysis based solely on their estimated proportion of ancestry, using the results from *Structure* or similar methods. We were unable to use this approach due to lack of high density SNP genotyping in the validation sample set. Interestingly, 8 out of 14 SNPs genotyped in the validation sample set had genotype distributions that significantly differed ($p>0.05$) between the non-Hispanic White and Hispanic White subgroups, and 12 out of the 14 SNPs had significantly different distributions between the non-Hispanic White and African American subgroups. While a large fraction of SNPs in the genome display differences in allele frequencies across racial subpopulations, this does reinforce the possibility of confounding due to stratification. The non-replication could also be due to unknown heterogeneity between the discovery and validation sample sets. This heterogeneity could be a clinical characteristic (e.g., depression subtype) or epistatic DNA variation that was not controlled for in the sample splitting, but that nonetheless alters the strength of the association. Genotype quality in the discovery set could also be a concern. We found two SNPs (rs4246510 and rs6489035) out of the 14 that we assayed using Taqman had genotype differences between Affymetrix's call and our Taqman data, with the other 12 SNPs having almost perfect concordance. Given the large amount of data to be scored, perfectly accurate genotyping cannot be expected in every case, and indeed, follow-up genotyping of the entire set using alternative methods will guard against false positive associations due to genotyping artifacts. However, false negative associations in the discovery set due to genotyping error will be harder to detect and perhaps more costly. Extending or altering the BRLMM algorithm, which is designed to give the highest call rates the data allows, to focus on call quality (and structural DNA variants, see below) will be useful and is under development (11).

As mentioned previously, this study was designed to investigate only the most "low hanging fruit", and was not intended to be a comprehensive follow-up of the discovery sample set results. Certainly, additional genetic models need to be tested in the discovery set (dominant, recessive, etc.). Also, a larger proportion of follow-up SNPs will need to be genotyped. This scale of genotyping would be best performed using highly multiplexed assays such as the MiP assay. Given the two-stage study design, multiple correction penalties for the follow-up of SNPs will be far less than the correction for the entire WGA panels, allowing for more liberal selection criteria. The statistical sacrifice with the two-stage design is of course a reduction in power. However, even with a split sample, we can capture (and replicate) clinically meaningful effect sizes with reasonable power. An FDR based approach may be worthwhile given that the actual causative SNPs may not be the most highly associated SNPs. Interestingly, applying an FDR approach to the data presented here reveals that only a single SNP (rs6489035) in the intolerance phenotype has a reasonable chance (q<0.10) of not being a false positive signal. However, this SNP did not replicate the association in the validation sample set, and in fact the directionality of the association changed between the two sample sets. Permutation techniques could also be used, but due to current computational limits, "stop points" for the analysis would have to be specified, though newer techniques can approximate permutation results more quickly (12). Alternatively, follow-up SNPs could also be selected using an effect-size (OR) threshold, instead of one based on an α threshold. This approach may be of particular utility in pharmacogenetic studies, where the eventual goal is to develop genetic tests for use in clinical treatment. Fine mapping of SNPs in the validation set for regions surrounding the putatively associated SNPs would also be beneficial, since differences in LD patterns across the discovery and validation sample sets could complicate indirect association analysis. Indirect association analysis could also possibly be improved through use of haplotype testing, with the hope of "tagging" untyped SNPs through use of multimarker haplotypes (13). However, the statistical penalties for multiple testing and the computational burden may limit the utility of haplotype analysis in WGA studies. Bayesian techniques, incorporating other SNP information (known functional change, conserved genomic region, expression changes, etc.) as weights in determining the ranking of follow-up SNPs could also be used (14). In addition to SNP data, the panels used to genotype the discovery sample set yield quantitative hybridization data that can in theory be used to score copy number variations, or CNVs (15). Identifying and testing these CNVs for association to citalopram response would be worthwhile, though the techniques for performing this are still being developed.

For complex genetic diseases, the common disease common variant hypothesis states that several DNA variants will, in combination, contribute a clinically meaningful risk of having the phenotype. Techniques for uncovering interacting loci are poorly developed, largely due to the computational and statistical burden of the number of tests that can be performed. For instance, performing all pairwise comparisons (SNP x SNP) with our WGA panels would require 1.7×10^{11} statistical tests. With this many tests needing correction, sample sizes like the one used in this study have power only to detect implausibly large interaction effects (16). The correction penalties for three and four way SNP interactions are even larger. Additionally, as higher level interaction testing is performed, the number of subjects with the causative allelic combination is reduced, further decreasing statistical power. Thus, for powerful interaction analysis, extremely large clinical populations will need to be collected. Here, we used decision trees as a way to test for interactions in a step-wise manner in order to avoid having to perform all pair-wise comparisons. Decision trees also have the added benefit of being easily interpreted. However, given the large number of possible trees, decision trees and related modeling methods have a tendency to over-fit the training set data. This is likely why our decision trees were not predictive in the validation sample set. Thus, replication of SNP interactions in different populations will be essential in association studies, as well as the development of powerful interaction testing strategies utilized on real data (17-19).

In summary, here we have presented the preliminary results of a two stage whole genome association study for citalopram remission and intolerance using the STAR*D clinical population. While none of the single locus associations (N=9) or SNP interaction decision trees in our discovery sample set met our strict replication criteria in the validation sample set, further genotyping and analysis is required to comprehensively follow-up the discovery set results. Given the lack of understanding of citalopram's mechanism of action, gene-agnostic studies such as these may be required to find genetic markers that are informative of remission or intolerance, if they exist.

6.5 References

1. Syvanen AC. Toward genome-wide SNP genotyping. *Nat Genet* 2005.

2. Klein RJ, Zeiss C, Chew EY, Tsai JY, Sackler RS, Haynes C, Henning AK, SanGiovanni JP, Mane SM, Mayne ST, Bracken MB, Ferris FL, Ott J, Barnstable C, Hoh J. Complement Factor H polymorphism in age-related macular degeneration. *Science* 2005; 308(5720):385-9.

3. Lawrence RW, Evans DM, Cardon LR. Prospects and pitfalls in whole genome association studies. *Philos Trans R Soc Lond B Biol Sci* 2005; 360(1460):1589-1595.

4. Tabor HK, Risch NJ, Myers RM. Opinion: Candidate-gene approaches for studying complex genetic traits: practical considerations. *Nat Rev Genet* 2002; 3(5):391-397.

5. Wang H, Thomas DC, Pe'er I, Stram DO. Optimal two-stage genotyping designs for genome-wide association scans. *Genet Epidemiol* 2006; 30(4):356-368.

6. Kennedy GC, Matsuzaki H, Dong S, Liu WM, Huang J, Liu G, Su X, Cao M, Chen W, Zhang J, Liu W, Yang G, Di X, Ryder T, He Z, Surti U, Phillips MS, Boyce-Jacino MT, Fodor SP, Jones KW. Large-scale genotyping of complex DNA. *Nat Biotech* 2003; 21(10):1233-1237.

7. Rabbee N, Speed TP. A genotype calling algorithm for affymetrix SNP arrays. *Bioinformatics* 2006; 22(1):7-12.

8. Hardenbol P, Baner J, Jain M, Nilsson M, Namsaraev EA, Karlin-Neumann GA, Fakhrai-Rad H, Ronaghi M, Willis TD, Landegren U, Davis RW. Multiplexed genotyping with sequence-tagged molecular inversion probes. *Nat Biotechnol* 2003; 21(6):673-678.

9.   Falush D, Stephens M, Pritchard JK. Inference of population structure using

multilocus genotype data: linked loci and correlated allele frequencies. *Genetics* 2003;

164(4):1567-1587.

10.   Skol AD, Scott LJ, Abecasis GR, Boehnke M. Joint analysis is more efficient

than replication-based analysis for two-stage genome-wide association studies. *Nat

Genet* 2006; 38(2):209-213.

11.   Hua J, Craig DW, Brun M, Webster J, Zismann V, Tembe W, Joshipura K,

Huentelman MJ, Dougherty ER, Stephan DA. SNiPer-HD: improved genotype calling

accuracy by an expectation-maximization algorithm for high-density SNP arrays.

Bioinformatics 2007; 23(1):57-63.

12.   Seaman SR, Muller-Myhsok B. Rapid simulation of p-values for product

methods and multiple-testing adjustment in association studies. *Am J Hum Genet*

2005; 76(3):399-408.

13.   Pe'er I, de Bakker PIW, Maller J, Yelensky R, Altshuler D, Daly MJ.

Evaluating and improving power in whole-genome association studies using fixed

marker sets. *Nat Genet* 2006; 38(6):663-667.

14.   Hoti F, Sillanpaa MJ. Bayesian mapping of genotype x expression interactions

in quantitative and qualitative traits. *Heredity* 2006; 97(1):4-18.

15.   Komura D, Shen F, Ishikawa S, Fitch KR, Chen W, Zhang J, Liu G, Ihara S,

Nakamura H, Hurles ME, Lee C, Scherer SW, Jones KW, Shapero MH, Huang J,

Aburatani H. Genome-wide detection of human copy number variations using high-

density DNA oligonucleotide arrays. *Genome Res* 2006; 16(12):1575-1584.

16.   Evans DM, Marchini J, Morris AP, Cardon LR. Two-stage two-locus models in

genome-wide association. *PLoS Genet* 2006; 2(9):e157.

17. Marchini J, Donnelly P, Cardon LR. Genome-wide strategies for detecting multiple loci that influence complex diseases. *Nat Genet* 2005; 37(4):413-417.

18. Kooperberg C, Bis JC, Marciante KD, Heckbert SR, Lumley T, Psaty BM. Logic regression for analysis of the association between genetic variation in the renin-angiotensin system and myocardial infarction or stroke. *Am J Epidemiol* 2006.

19. Kooperberg C, Ruczinski I. Identifying interacting SNPs using Monte Carlo logic regression. *Genet Epidemiol* 2005; 28(2):157-170.

CHAPTER 7

SUMMARY AND FUTURE DIRECTIONS

7.1 Summary of thesis

The experiments described in the previous chapters have attempted to establish genetic markers that are predictive of a depressed subject's clinical outcome following antidepressant therapy. To that end, several complementary genetic approaches have been utilized (outlined in Figure 1.1). Our initial efforts focused on linkage disequilibrium (LD) mapping of several serotonin-related pharmacodynamic candidate genes (*HTR1A*, *HTR2A*, *HTR2C*, *TPH1*, *TPH2*, and *MAOA*) using 110 SNPs selected from the online database dbSNP. In a small but highly characterized (N=96) depressed patient population taking the selective serotonin reuptake inhibitor (SSRI) fluoxetine, several SNPs and multimarker haplotypes in these genes were associated (p<0.05) with response and response specificity (1). In order to uncover novel tagSNPs or potentially functional variants, the coding regions, intron-exon boundaries, and conserved non-coding regions were directly sequenced in all subjects in the fluoxetine population. While no obvious functional variants were discovered in these genes, a few additional tagSNPs were identified, which provide more comprehensive coverage of the variation in these regions. In an attempt to replicate the initial associations, the tagSNPs were then genotyped in the large STAR*D population (N=1,953), which had been given the SSRI citalopram. None of the variants were associated with citalopram response or response specificity. This non-replication could be due to several factors including simple Type I error, differences between the drug's mechanism of action, or unknown differences between the clinical populations.

218

We then explored pharmacokinetic gene variation as a possible modulator of citalopram response or tolerance. Instead of the indirect LD based approach we used for the pharmacodynamic candidate genes, here we utilized a direct association approach since there are known, functional variants in several relevant pharmacokinetic genes (*ABCB1*, *CYP3A4*, *CYP3A5*, *CYP2C19*, and *CYP2D6*). Using a two-stage study design, none of the pharmacokinetic variants that we screened in the STAR*D population were significantly ($p<0.05$) associated with citalopram response or tolerance in both the discovery and validation sample sets.

Given the difficulty in predicting relevant candidate genes *a priori*, we used a whole genome association (WGA) platform and a two-stage study design to genotype over 590,000 SNPs in approximately half of the STAR*D sample. Several of these SNPs were associated with citalopram remission and tolerance at a very high significance level in the discovery sample set. We attempted to replicate the nine most significantly associated SNPs in the validation sample set. However, none of the SNPs showed significant ($p<0.05$) association with remission or tolerance in the validation sample set. Furthermore, the multi-SNP decision trees that were constructed using the discovery sample dataset were not predictive of remission or tolerance using the validation sample set SNP data. This non-replication could be due to a variety of factors, including uncorrected population stratification, unknown clinical confounders, or simple Type I error in the discovery set. However, this was an attempt to replicate the "low hanging fruit" of the discovery portion of the WGA study. For example, the "truly" associated variants may not have provided the most extreme estimates of statistical significance, and instead may be represented by more modest, but consistent, measures of significance. The most extreme values may be enriched with signals due to the factors listed above and others, such as genotyping errors. An unanswered question is how far to pursue findings for replication (e.g., absolute p-value threshold, effect size, significance in more than one subgroup of phenotype). In order to fully explore the initial discovery set findings, much more genotyping of the validation set will need to be performed. This will allow additional analytical techniques, such as different genetic models, the ability to control for stratification in the validation set, and more rigorous testing of variant interactions, all of which will be important to comprehensively explore the role of genetic variation in SSRI response.

7.2 Future directions

The field of complex human phenotype genetics has been evolving at an amazing pace since the sequencing of the human genome. Much of the evolution of the field can be traced to rapidly advancing genotyping technologies that increase genotype throughput and reduce genotyping costs. For instance, when this project was started in 2002, most genetic association studies investigated less than a dozen candidate SNPs, with most focusing on a single marker. Our initial fluoxetine pharmacodynamic gene project involving 110 SNPs was considered a formidable amount of genotyping at the time and the genotyping took approximately 4 months to complete. With current multiplex technologies, such as Illumina's BeadArray assay (2), the genotyping would require less than a week of laboratory work and could genotype many more SNPs (3). Larger scale genotyping, like our WGA study involving 590,000 SNPs, can now be completed in a few weeks. The scale of genotyping will continue to grow, as Affymetrix and Illumina have both already announced the commercialization of a 1 million SNP panel, part of which will be designed to detect copy number variants (CNVs). It is now becoming clear that within the next decade, whole genome resequencing of large sample sets will become economically feasible. A question with both practical and theoretical implications, however, is will the field be able to interpret such high density genetic data?

Analytical techniques in complex phenotype genetics have not evolved as quickly as methods for genotyping. For instance, around 10 years ago, it was still unclear whether useful amounts of LD exist in the human genome (4). It is clear now that significant LD extends to useful distances in outbred human populations (5;6). At the time of our initial fluoxetine pharmacodynamic project, it was still necessary to empirically measure LD in a region of interest. Our work showed these serotonin-related genes to have extensive LD, which was not a foregone conclusion at the time. Unfortunately, this LD resulted in redundancy in our genotyping. The international HapMap project, which was completed (phase II) after this project, allows users to select tagging SNPs from the publicly avaiable dataset of dense markers across the genome, which is an invaluable resource to LD mapping. However, much is still unclear about the most powerful way to utilize LD in association studies. For instance, the use of haplotypes in association studies needs further development (7). When this project was started, techniques for inferring haplotypes from unphased genotype data and testing for association were in their infancy (8). Currently, the utility of haplotype testing in association studies is still debatable, as some feel it does not add enough additional information to single locus testing to justify the multiple correction penalties (9). A substantial number of methods have been published in the past five years that utilize LD in order to select tagging SNPs (10-14). It seems that the most analytically straightforward, based on a threshold for pairwise r^2, has also become the most popular method for selecting tagging SNPs, though other methods appear to be more efficient at reducing genotyping load. It's still unclear exactly how well tagging SNPs will transfer across different human populations, although much research has focused on this question (15;16). These may ultimately be moot considerations, given that whole genome resequencing will soon make tagging unnecessary.

One of the major hurdles in the development of analytical methods is the issue of multiple testing (17). It is difficult to separate true associations from those caused by chance when performing 500,000 or more single locus tests. When several phenotypes and several populations are examined, the problem obviously is amplified. The problem becomes much larger when searching for interacting SNPs, which are a cornerstone of the common disease common variant hypothesis. False discovery rate (FDR) methods can be used to gauge how many SNPs to move forward in multi-stage studies, and aren't affected by inter-marker relatedness (18). Increases in computational power will allow for permutation based methods to be applied across entire WGA panels, which will take into account inter-marker relatedness. Bayesian methodology, incorporating information from QTLs, multi-species alignments, or functional predictions may also be useful (19). However, given the inherent risk of Type I error from the number of tests and since we often have no *a priori* reason to believe putatively associated SNPs in WGA studies, replication in separate populations will be of paramount importance. Even this gold standard is problematic, when "independent" populations may differ subtly by phenotypic definition or less subtly by differences in population ancestry or genotyping platform. Statistical limits may make innovative study designs, along with the collection of large clinical populations for replication, the only way to get through the multiple testing concerns in large scale associations studies.

Another key to the success of future large scale association studies will be the development of statistically powerful techniques for uncovering interacting SNPs. The common disease common variant (CDCV) hypothesis predicts that individual variants will have small phenotypic effect sizes (20). However, in combination, variants are thought to have clinically meaningful effects, although there are few examples of such interactions (21;22). In our studies we attempted to find variant interactions using logistic regression (for small numbers of SNPs) and decision trees (for the WGA data). While neither of these techniques uncovered significantly interacting SNPs in our data, they may have utility in other studies. However, one particular barrier for the development of interacting SNPs models is the multiple testing burden (which increases exponentially with the number of SNPs investigated); additionally, power is further reduced by the limited number of subjects with each causative allelic combination. The collection of large clinical samples is the only way to overcome these statistical limits. Once interacting SNPs have been discovered and validated in these large sample collections, easily interpretable clinical diagnostic models will also need to be developed. However, pharmacogenetic models that are limited to using only genetic markers for association to clinical outcome may not be capturing a large portion of the variation in response. Robust clinical models for personalized medicine will require non-genetic biomarkers (e.g., protein expression, liver function tests, etc.) as well as clinical demographics (age, concomitant medications, race, etc.) in order to have maximum utility. Pharmacogenetic phenotypes, as opposed to most complex disease phenotypes, have the additional benefit of allowing for alteration of pharmacological treatment once susceptibility variants and other factors are known.

A major concern for population based association studies has been the risk of confounding due to population stratification. Population stratification is thought to play a role in the non-replication of many association studies, and as study populations become larger the risk of confounding also increases. Current methods for detecting and correcting for population stratification, such as *structure*, can perform adequately, but for small scale genotyping studies they require additional marker genotyping which can be cost prohibitive (23). The development of efficient ancestry informative marker (AIM) panels that have maximal allele frequency differences across subpopulations would have great utility in small scale association studies. The selection of AIMs for distant subpopulations (e.g., Africans and Asians) in order to detect large levels of stratification is straightforward, given the dense marker data available from the HapMap project (24-26). Recent reports suggest population stratification may have a confounding effect even within isolated populations such as Iceland and Europe, which were both thought to be relatively homogeneous (27;28). Selection of AIMs for more subtle levels of stratification across continental clines will require more large scale genotyping in these subpopulations in order to define their allele frequencies. For WGA studies, and in the future whole genome resequencing studies, the dense amount of marker data available should allow for accurate matching of cases and control based on ancestry and consequently little reduction in statistical power.

Single nucleotide polymorphisms have been the workhorse of genetic association studies for the past decade, largely because of their ability to be easily assayed in a cost-effective manner. However, it is becoming clear that other types of variation, namely copy number variation (CNVs), is common in the genome and may contribute to human phenotypes. Copy number variants take the form of segmental duplications or deletions, and are thought to alter at least as much of the human genome as SNPs (29). Given their sizable changes to the genome, CNVs are reasonably thought to cause considerable differences in expression or function of the genes they encompass, although there is little evidence for this as of yet. Since the majority of genotyping techniques focus on a small area around the SNP of interest (generally less than 100 bp), CNVs that encompass interrogated SNPs can have a detrimental and often unknown effect on genotype accuracy and quality. Fortunately in WGA studies, current genotyping methods often rely on hybridization to a fixed DNA array, which yields quantitative data and thus can be scored for copy number variants as well as SNPs (30). Currently limiting the widespread utilization of CNVs in WGA studies are efficient algorithms for scoring them from the raw genotype data as well as a catalog of common CNVs in the human genome, which would help by narrowing the search space. A large, detailed search for common CNVs across the genome similar to the SNP Consortium project would greatly aid in the integration of CNVs into WGA studies.

As was mentioned above, large collections of well-phenotyped subjects is crucial to the success of pharmacogenetics in the next decade. Large populations are necessary in order to provide replication of initial findings, to lessen the multiple testing burden by increasing power, and for studies of interacting SNPs, which is a crux of the common disease common variant hypothesis of complex diseases. Alternatively, for the common disease rare variant hypothesis, where individual variants are thought to have large effect sizes but occur very infrequently, large collections of patients will be necessary to find adequate number of subjects carrying the risk variant. Single investigators typically have the resources to collect on the order of hundreds of patients at best. Large government sponsored clinical trials (such as STAR*D) and late phase investigational drug trials can involve large numbers of subjects, but usually not more than two or three thousand. Even with all the resources used to fund such studies, sufficiently powered pharmacogenetic studies will require many more, on the order of tens of thousands of patients. For this scale of populations, large consortia will need to be formed, where investigators share subject DNA, phenotype data, and ultimately, credit for any findings. An example of an effort on a similar scale can be seen with the Type I diabetes genetic consortium (31). Having the foresight to collect DNA from all consenting individuals enrolled in a large Phase 3 drug trial will hopefully become more common as the field develops. The use of large health insurance registries (such as Kaiser Permanente in California) could aid in identifying subjects, but could prove complicated due to their retrospective nature. As academic medical centers (such as UCSF) and large hospitals move towards fully electronic record keeping, enrolling patients (and collecting DNA) at admittance or discharge for pharmacogenetic studies of common medications may be a realistic way of enrolling large numbers of subjects. As with all epidemiological research, false positive and dashed hopes are common, and more subjects are always needed. I feel with cooperation among researches, adequate resources, hard work and a little luck, in the next ten years there will be profound examples of the clinical utility of prescribing the right drug to the right person at the right time and dose.

7.3 References

1.   Peters EJ, Slager SL, McGrath PJ, Knowles JA, Hamilton SP. Investigation of serotonin-related genes in antidepressant response. *Mol Psychiatry* 2004; 9(9):879-889.

2.   Fan JB, Hu SX, Craumer WC, Barker DL. BeadArray-based solutions for enabling the promise of pharmacogenomics. *Biotechniques* 2005; 39(4):583-588.

3.   Liu ET. New technologies for high-throughput analysis. *Pharmacogenomics* 2005; 6(5):469-471.

4.   Huttley GA, Smith MW, Carrington M, O'Brien SJ. A scan for linkage disequilibrium across the human genome. *Genetics* 1999; 152(4):1711-1722.

5.   Reich DE, Cargill M, Bolk S, Ireland J, Sabeti PC, Richter DJ, Lavery T, Kouyoumjian R, Farhadian SF, Ward R, Lander ES. Linkage disequilibrium in the human genome. *Nature* 2001; 411(6834):199-204.

6.   Ardlie KG, Kruglyak L, Seielstad M. Patterns of linkage disequilibrium in the human genome. *Nat Rev Genet* 2002; 3(4):299-309.

7.   Schaid DJ. Evaluating associations of haplotypes with traits. *Genet Epidemiol* 2004; 27(4):348-364.

8.   Stephens M, Smith NJ, Donnelly P. A new statistical method for haplotype reconstruction from population data. *Am J Hum Genet* 2001; 68(4):978-989.

9.   Clark AG. The role of haplotypes in candidate gene studies. *Genet Epidemiol* 2004; 27(4):321-333.

10.   Carlson CS, Eberle MA, Rieder MJ, Yi Q, Kruglyak L, Nickerson DA. Selecting a maximally informative set of single-nucleotide polymorphisms for association analyses using linkage disequilibrium. *Am J Hum Genet* 2004; 74(1):106-120.

11. Weale ME, Depondt C, Macdonald SJ, Smith A, Lai PS, Shorvon SD, Wood NW, Goldstein DB. Selection and evaluation of tagging SNPs in the neuronal-sodium-channel gene SCN1A: implications for linkage-disequilibrium gene mapping. *Am J Hum Genet* 2003; 73(3):551-565.

12. Ke X, Cardon LR. Efficient selective screening of haplotype tag SNPs. *Bioinformatics* 2003; 19(2):287-288.

13. Stram DO. Tag SNP selection for association studies. *Genet Epidemiol* 2004.

14. Liu Z, Lin S, Tan M. Genome-wide tagging SNPs with entropy-based Monte Carlo method. *J Comput Biol* 2006; 13(9):1606-1614.

15. De Bakker PI, Burtt NP, Graham RR, Guiducci C, Yelensky R, Drake JA, Bersaglieri T, Penney KL, Butler J, Young S, Onofrio RC, Lyon HN, Stram DO, Haiman CA, Freedman ML, Zhu X, Cooper R, Groop L, Kolonel LN, Henderson BE, Daly MJ, Hirschhorn JN, Altshuler D. Transferability of tag SNPs in genetic association studies in multiple populations. *Nat Genet* 2006; 38(11):1298-1303.

16. Mueller JC, Lohmussaar E, Magi R, Remm M, Bettecken T, Lichtner P, Biskup S, Illig T, Pfeufer A, Luedemann J, Schreiber S, Pramstaller P, Pichler I, Romeo G, Gaddi A, Testa A, Wichmann HE, Metspalu A, Meitinger T. Linkage disequilibrium patterns and tagSNP transferability among European populations. *Am J Hum Genet* 2005; 76(3):387-398.

17. Carlson CS, Eberle MA, Kruglyak L, Nickerson DA. Mapping complex disease loci in whole-genome association studies. *Nature* 2004; 429(6990):446-452.

18. Fernando RL, Nettleton D, Southey BR, Dekkers JC, Rothschild MF, Soller M. Controlling the proportion of false positives in multiple dependent tests. *Genetics* 2004; 166(1):611-619.

19.   Rannala B. Finding genes influencing susceptibility to complex diseases in the post-genome era. *Am J Pharmacogenomics* 2001; 1(3):203-221.

20.   Mayeux R. Mapping the new frontier: complex genetic disorders. *J Clin Invest* 2005; 115(6):1404-1407.

21.   Chumakov I, Blumenfeld M, Guerassimenko O, Cavarec L, Palicio M, Abderrahim H, Bougueleret L, Barry C, Tanaka H, La Rosa P, Puech A, Tahri N, Cohen-Akenine A, Delabrosse S, Lissarrague S, Picard FP, Maurice K, Essioux L, Millasseau P, Grel P, Debailleul V, Simon AM, Caterina D, Dufaure I, Malekzadeh K, Belova M, Luan JJ, Bouillot M, Sambucy JL, Primas G, Saumier M, Boubkiri N, Martin-Saumier S, Nasroune M, Peixoto H, Delaye A, Pinchot V, Bastucci M, Guillou S, Chevillon M, Sainz-Fuertes R, Meguenni S, Aurich-Costa J, Cherif D, Gimalac A, Van Duijn C, Gauvreau D, Ouellette G, Fortier I, Raelson J, Sherbatich T, Riazanskaia N, Rogaev E, Raeymaekers P, Aerssens J, Konings F, Luyten W, Macciardi F, Sham PC, Straub RE, Weinberger DR, Cohen N, Cohen D, Ouelette G, Realson J. Genetic and physiological data implicating the new human gene G72 and the gene for D-amino acid oxidase in schizophrenia. *Proc Natl Acad Sci U S A* 2002; 99(21):13675-13680.

22.   Stoll M, Corneliussen B, Costello CM, Waetzig GH, Mellgard B, Koch WA, Rosenstiel P, Albrecht M, Croucher PJ, Seegert D, Nikolaus S, Hampe J, Lengauer T, Pierrou S, Foelsch UR, Mathew CG, Lagerstrom-Fermer M, Schreiber S. Genetic variation in DLG5 is associated with inflammatory bowel disease. *Nat Genet* 2004; 36(5):476-480.

23.   Falush D, Stephens M, Pritchard JK. Inference of Population Structure Using Multilocus Genotype Data. Linked loci and correlated allele frequencies. *Genetics* 2003; 164(4):1567-1587.

24.   Choudhry S, Coyle N, Tang H, Salari K, Lind D, Clark S, Tsai HJ, Naqvi M,

Phong A, Ung N, Matallana H, Avila P, Casal J, Torres A, Nazario S, Castro R, Battle

N, Perez-Stable E, Kwok PY, Sheppard D, Shriver M, Rodriguez-Cintron W, Risch

N, Ziv E, Burchard E, Genetics of Asthma in Latino Americans (GALA) Study.

Population stratification confounds genetic association studies among Latinos. *Hum

Genet* 2006; 118(5):652-664.

25.   Seldin MF, Shigeta R, Villoslada P, Selmi C, Tuomilehto J, Silva G, Belmont

JW, Klareskog L, Gregersen PK. European population substructure: clustering of

northern and southern populations. *PLoS Genet* 2006; 2(9):e143.

26.   Tian C, Hinds DA, Shigeta R, Kittles R, Ballinger DG, Seldin MF. A

genomewide single-nucleotide-polymorphism panel with high ancestry information

for African American admixture mapping. *Am J Hum Genet* 2006; 79(4):640-649.

27.   Helgason A, Yngvadottir B, Hrafnkelsson B, Gulcher J, Stefansson K. An

Icelandic example of the impact of population structure on association studies. *Nat

Genet* 2005; 37(1):90-95.

28.   Campbell CD, Ogburn EL, Lunetta KL, Lyon HN, Freedman ML, Groop LC,

Altshuler D, Ardlie KG, Hirschhorn JN. Demonstrating stratification in a European

American population. *Nat Genet* 2005; 37(8):868-872.

29.   Redon R, Ishikawa S, Fitch KR, Feuk L, Perry GH, Andrews TD, Fiegler H,

Shapero MH, Carson AR, Chen W, Cho EK, Dallaire S, Freeman JL, Gonzalez JR,

Gratacos M, Huang J, Kalaitzopoulos D, Komura D, MacDonald JR, Marshall CR,

Mei R, Montgomery L, Nishimura K, Okamura K, Shen F, Somerville MJ, Tchinda J,

Valsesia A, Woodwark C, Yang F, Zhang J, Zerjal T, Zhang J, Armengol L, Conrad

DF, Estivill X, Tyler-Smith C, Carter NP, Aburatani H, Lee C, Jones KW, Scherer

SW, Hurles ME. Global variation in copy number in the human genome. *Nature* 2006; 444(7118):444-454.

30.   Carson AR, Feuk L, Mohammed M, Scherer SW. Strategies for the detection of copy number and other structural variants in the human genome. *Hum Genomics* 2006; 2(6):403-414.

31.   Rich SS, Concannon P, Erlich H, Julier C, Morahan G, Nerup J, Pociot F, Todd JA. The Type 1 Diabetes Genetics Consortium. *Ann N Y Acad Sci* 2006; 10791-8.

www.ingramcontent.com/pod-product-compliance
Lightning Source LLC
Chambersburg PA
CBHW060357220326
41598CB00023B/2944